Pulmonary Cytopathology

ESSENTIALS IN CYTOPATHOLOGY SERIES

Dorothy L. Rosenthal, MD, FIAC, Series Editor

Editorial Board
Syed Z. Ali, MD
Douglas P. Clark, MD
Yener S. Erozan, MD

---

1. D.P. Clark and W.C. Faquin: Thyroid Cytopathology. 2005
ISBN 0-387-23304-0

2. D.L. Rosenthal and S.S. Raab: Cytologic Detection of Urothelial Lesions. 2005
ISBN 0-387-23945-6

3. D.C. Chhieng and E.B. Stelow: Pancreatic Cytopathology. 2007
ISBN 978-0-387-68946-3

4. S.Z. Ali and A.V. Parwani: Breast Cytopathology. 2007
ISBN 978-0-387-71594-0

5. W.C. Faquin and C.N. Powers: Salivary Gland Cytopathology. 2008
ISBN 978-0-387-76622-5

6. Y.S. Erozan and I. Ramzy: Pulmonary Cytopathology. 2009
ISBN 978-0-387-88886-6

Yener S. Erozan, MD

Department of Pathology, Johns Hopkins School of Medicine,
Baltimore, Maryland

Ibrahim Ramzy, MD

Departments of Pathology-Laboratory Medicine
& Obstetrics-Gynecology, University of California Irvine,
Irvine, California

Pulmonary Cytopathology

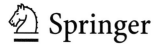

Yener S. Erozan, MD
Professor of Pathology
The Johns Hopkins School
    of Medicine
Baltimore, MD 21287, USA
yerozan@jhmi.edu

Ibrahim Ramzy, MD
Professor of Pathology-Laboratory
Medicine & Obstetrics-Gynecology
University of California Irvine
Irvine, CA 92697, USA
iramzy@uci.edu

Series Editor
Dorothy L. Rosenthal, MD, FIAC
Professor of Pathology, Oncology and Gynecology/Obstetrics
The Johns Hopkins School of Medicine
Baltimore, MD 21287, USA

ISBN 978-0-387-88886-6   e-ISBN 978-0-387-88888-0
DOI 10.1007/978-0-387-88888-0

Library of Congress Control Number: 2008940854

Series Preface

The subspecialty of Cytopathology is 60 years old and has become established as a solid and reliable discipline in medicine. As expected, cytopathology literature has expanded in a remarkably short period of time, from a few textbooks prior to the 1980s to a current library of texts and journals devoted exclusively to cytomorphology that is substantial. *Essentials in Cytopathology* does not presume to replace any of the distinguished textbooks in Cytopathology. Instead, the series will publish generously illustrated and user-friendly guides for both pathologists and clinicians.

Building on the amazing success of *The Bethesda System for Reporting Cervical Cytology,* now in its second edition, the *Series* will utilize a similar format including minimal text, tabular criteria and superb illustrations based on real-life specimens. *Essentials in Cytopathology* will, at times, deviate from the classic organization of pathology texts. The logic of decision trees, elimination of unlikely choices and narrowing of differential diagnosis via a pragmatic approach based on morphologic criteria will be some of the strategies used to illustrate principles and practice in Cytopathology.

Most of the authors for *Essentials in Cytopathology* are faculty members in The Johns Hopkins University School of Medicine, Department of Pathology, Division of Cytopathology. They bring to each volume the legacy of John K. Frost and the collective experience of a preeminent cytopathology service. The archives at Hopkins are meticulously catalogued and form the framework for text and illustrations. Authors from other institutions have been selected on the basis of their national reputations, experience and enthusiasm for Cytopathology. They bring to the series complimentary viewpoints and enlarge the scope of materials contained in the photographs.

The editor and authors are indebted to our students, past and future, who challenge and motivate us to become the best that we possibly can be. We share that experience with you through these pages, and hope that you will learn from them as we have from those who have come before us. We would be remiss if we did not pay tribute to our professional colleagues, the cytotechnologists and preparatory technicians who lovingly care for the specimens that our clinical colleagues send to us.

And finally, we cannot emphasize enough throughout these volumes the importance of collaboration with the patient care team. Every specimen comes to us as a question begging an answer. Without input from the clinicians, complete patient history, results of imaging studies and other ancillary tests, we cannot perform optimally. It is our responsibility to educate our clinicians about their role in our interpretation, and for us to integrate as much information as we can gather into our final diagnosis, even if the answer at first seems obvious.

We hope you will find this series useful and welcome your feedback as you place these handbooks by your microscopes, and into your bookbags.

Baltimore, Maryland   Dorothy L. Rosenthal, M.D., FIAC
July 15, 2004

Contents

Introduction

Pulmonary cytopathology comprises a significant proportion of the non-gynecologic cytopathology practice in hospital-based laboratories. Development of advanced radiological techniques have improved the detection of and access to smaller lesions of the lung, at the same time creating new challenges for the radiologist and pathologist to obtain representative specimens from the lesion and establish a diagnosis on limited cytologic and histologic specimens. Rapidly expanding applications of immunohistochemistry and immunocytochemistry on cytologic (smears, cytospins, and liquid preparations) and histologic (e.g., cell blocks and core biopsies) preparations, help to determine the origin and nature of lesions; but have added new challenges for pathologists who must make prudent choices about these techniques and then interpret the results in correlation with morphologic findings.

In this book, the characteristic cytologic features as well as the spectrum of changes in selected benign lesions and malignant neoplasms will be presented, along with the appropriate use of ancillary techniques to aid in the diagnosis. Emphasis will be placed on differential diagnosis between benign and malignant diseases and among the various types of neoplasms.

Chapter 1
Specimen Collection and Processing

Proper collection and processing of cytologic specimens are crucial for an accurate cytopathologic diagnosis. In most instances, failure to establish a definitive diagnosis is caused either by inadequate sampling of the lesion or by suboptimal preparation of the specimen.

Specimen Collection

Pulmonary specimen collection techniques are listed in Table 1.1. The most frequently used techniques in current practice are bronchoscopy and fine needle aspiration (FNA). FNAs (transbronchial or transthoracic) are performed under imaging guidance, i.e., ultrasound (US) or computed tomography (CT). More recently, EUS guided FNA is increasingly used in the diagnosis of mediastinal lesions and the staging of lung cancer. On-site evaluation for adequacy improves the yield of diagnosis in FNA. Selection of the technique is determined by the location of the lesion (Table 1.2) and also the expertise of the physician (e.g., radiologist, pulmonologist) performing the procedure.

Sputum

Early morning sputum, collected for three consecutive days when the patient wakes in the morning, gives the best results. The

Y.S. Erozan, I. Ramzy, *Pulmonary Cytopathology*,
Essentials in Cytopathology 6, DOI 10.1007/978-0-387-88888-0_1,
© Springer Science+Business Media, LLC 2009

Table 1.1 Pulmonary specimen collection techniques

Sputum
- Spontaneous (Early morning sputum, ×3)
- Induced

Bronchoscopic specimens
- Brushing
- Wash/aspirate
- Bronchoalveolar lavage (BAL)
- Transbronchial/tracheal FNA

Endoscopic ultrasound-guided (EUS) FNA
- Transtracheal/bronchial
- Transesophageal

Transthoracic (percutaneous) FNA

Table 1.2 Efficacy of specimen collection techniques according to location of lesion

Location	Effective technique
Proximal mucosal surface	Sputum, bronchial brush, bronchial wash
Proximal submucosal	Transbronchial/tracheal FNA
Peripheral	Transcutaneous FNA, bronchial brush, bronchoalveolar lavage
Peribronchial/tracheal/carinal	Transbronchial/tracheal FNA
Mediastinal	Transbronchial/tracheal, transcutaneous or endoscopic ultrasound–guided FNA

patient should be instructed to clear the throat, rinse the mouth, and cough deeply using the diaphragm. For induction, aerosol of heated hypertonic saline (10–15%) with 20% polypropylene glycol is inhaled. The specimens can be sent to the laboratory unfixed (if no significant delay is expected) or in an appropriate fixative or preservative such as Saccomanno solution.

Bronchoscopy Specimens

Bronchial Brush

The specimen is collected by brushing the suspected area under direct visualization or, without visualization, inserting the brush into smaller bronchi leading to the area where the lesion is located.

If direct smears from the brush are made, *immediate fixation in 70% ethyl alcohol is necessary* for optimal preservation of cellular features, which is crucial for accurate cytologic evaluation. Otherwise, the brush can be rinsed with a physiological solution [e.g., Hanks Balanced Salt Solution®] and sent to the laboratory.

Bronchial Wash/Aspirate

Aspirates of bronchial secretions and bronchial washes with normal saline are collected, usually following the brush. The material should be submitted to the laboratory for processing as quickly as possible to avoid any deterioration and loss of cytologic detail.

Bronchoalveolar Lavage (BAL)

This is performed by inserting the bronchoscope into the selected segment of bronchus until it is wedged, injecting 100–300 mL of normal saline, and aspirating 20- to 50-mL aliquots, thereby providing cellular samples from both bronchioles and alveoli.

Transbronchial/Tracheal FNAs

A flexible needle, introduced through a channel of a flexible bronchoscope, is inserted into the suspected area through the tracheal or bronchial wall. The lesion is aspirated, the needle withdrawn and the material submitted for examination. At on-site evaluation, two direct smears are prepared; one is immediately fixed in alcohol and the other is air-dried and stained with one of the Romanowsky stains (e.g. Diff-Quik) for on-site examination. The remaining material is rinsed with physiological solution (e.g., Hanks balanced salt solution) and sent to the laboratory for processing according to the laboratory's protocol. Whenever possible, cell blocks are prepared.

Transthoracic (Percutaneous) FNAs

This is performed under ultrasound (subpleural lesions) or CT guidance, using a 22 gauge or thinner needle. For core biopsies, a

20 gauge needle is used. In the co-axial biopsy method, a 20 gauge needle for core biopsy or thinner needle for fine needle aspiration is inserted through a 19 gauge needle. Sampling by fine needle can be done by moving the needle back and forth without aspiration (preferred method in our institution) or with aspiration if the lesion is sclerotic. The specimen is handled the same way as are the transbronchial FNAs. If core biopsies are obtained, they are fixed in formalin for tissue processing.

Processing Pulmonary Specimens

Sputum

Direct smears from unfixed specimens or concentration/homogenization techniques (e.g., Saccomanno technique) can be used.

Bronchial Brush, Wash, and BAL Specimens

These are usually processed according to the laboratory's liquid specimen procedures. Cytospins and other liquid media processing methods (e.g., ThinPrep, SurePath), with or without cell blocks, are used.

Staining

Papanicolaou stain is used for cytologic preparations of pulmonary specimens. Air-dried smears, as in on-site evaluation, are stained with Diff-Quik. Hematoxylin-Eosin (H&E) is the standard stain for histologic preparations (i.e., cell blocks, core biopsies). Special stains include those for acid-fast bacilli (e.g., Fite, Ziehl-Nielson) and fungi (PAS, GMS). Mucin stains (e.g., mucicarmine) and a large variety of immunostains are used to determine the type or origin of neoplasms in pulmonary specimens. Although these stains can be performed on smears or liquid-based preparations, the best results, specifically for immunostains, are obtained in histologic preparations, such as cell blocks or core biopsies.

Assessment of Specimen Adequacy

Assessment of adequacy of the sample is a prerequisite for reducing the incidence of false results, particularly false negatives. The criteria vary with the type of specimen procured. An adequate sputum specimen should include pulmonary macrophages (Fig.1.1A&B) and a few ciliated columnar cells. When present, Curschmann spirals are also indicative of deep pulmonary sample (Fig. 1.1 C). Specimens with abundant benign squamous cells are usually the result of oral contamination and should not be considered adequate. On the other hand, an abundance of ciliated

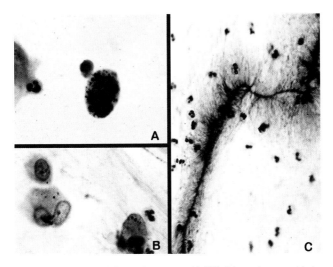

Fig. 1.1 Adequate (satisfactory) sputum. (**A&B**) Macrophages with intra-cytoplasmic carbon particles. (**C**) Curschmann spiral. These form in the small bronchi in conditions associated with peripheral airway constriction and increased mucus secretion. They are not infrequently seen in the sputum samples of smokers (Papanicolaou stain, high power)

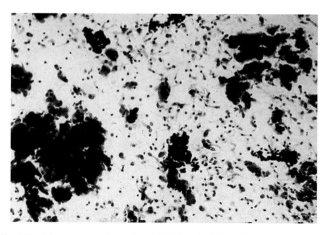

Fig. 1.2 Adequate specimen. Bronchial brush. Many tissue fragments and single cells of respiratory epithelium (Papanicolaou stain, low power)

columnar cells is a requirement for a bronchial brush or lavage to be considered as adequate (Fig. 1.2). An adequate bronchoalveolar lavage should contain a large number of pulmonary macrophages (Fig. 1.3), thus reflecting sampling of distal alveolar spaces and bronchioles.

In FNA specimens, ciliated columnar cells are usually encountered in endoscopic endobronchial procedures, but are lacking in percutaneous FNA specimens which are procured from more peripheral lesions. On-site evaluation for adequacy at the time of any FNA procedure offers major advantages to the patient, and immediate microscopic examination is now a common practice performed by the cytopathologist and cytotechnologist. Such rapid assessment increases the diagnostic yield and decreases the number of passes required for diagnosis, thus reducing discomfort and morbidity to the patient. The availability of on-site assessment also helps in deciding the appropriate allocation of specimens for special studies (e.g., flow cytometry, microbiological studies) and whether histologic preparations (i.e., cell block, additional core biopsy) are needed.

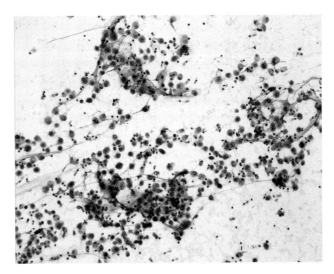

Fig. 1.3 Adequate specimen. Bronchoalveolar lavage (BAL). Many alveolar macrophages (Papanicolaou stain, low power)

Suggested Reading

Baker JJ, Solanki PH, Schenk DA, et al. Transbronchial fine needle aspiration of the mediastinum: importance of lymphocytes as an indicator of specimen adequacy. Acta Cytol 1990;3:517–523

Cham MD, Lane ME, Henschke CI, Yankelevitz DF. Lung biopsy: special techniques. Semin Respir Crit Care Med 2008 Aug;29(4):335–349

Chamberlain DW, Braude AC, Rebuck AS. A critical evaluation of bronchoalveolar lavage: criteria for identifying unsatisfactory specimens. Acta Cytol 1987;31:599–605

Choi Y-D, Han C-W, Kim J-H, et al. Effectiveness of sputum cytology using ThinPrep® method for evaluation of lung cancer. Diagn Cytopathol 2008;36:167–171

Dabbs DJ. Diagnostic immunohistochemistry, edn 2, Philadelphia, PA, Churchill Livingstone, 2006

Fischler DF, Toddy SM. Non-gynecologic cytology utilizing the ThinPrep processor. Acta Cytol 1996;40:669–675

Fraire AE, Underwood RD, McLarty JW, et al. Conventional respiratory cytology versus fine needle aspiration cytology in the diagnosis of lung cancer. Acta Cytol 1991;35:385–388

Garg S, Handa U, Mohan H, et al. Comparative analysis of various cyto-histological techniques in diagnosis of lung diseases. Diagn Cytopathol 2007;35:26–31

Hawes RH, Gress F, Kesler KA, et al. Endoscopic ultrasound versus computed tomography in the evaluation of the mediastinum in patients with non-small cell lung cancer. Endoscopy 1994;26:784–787

Layfield L, Coogan A, Johnson WW, et al. Transthoracic fine needle aspiration biopsy: sensitivity in relation to guidance technique and lesion size and location. Acta Cytol 1996;40:687–690

Linder J, Rennard SI. Bronchoalveolar lavage. Chicago, ASCP Press, 1988

Rivera MP, Mehta AC. Initial diagnosis of lung cancer. ACCP Evidence-based Clinical Practice Guideline (2nd edn). Chest 2007;132: 131S–148S

Rowe LR, Mulvihill SJ, Emerson L et al. Subcutaneous tumor seeding following needle core biopsy of hepatocellular carcinoma. Diagn Cytopathol 2007;35:717–721

Savoy AD, Ravenel JG, Hoffman BJ, et al. Endoscopic ultrasound for thoracic malignancy: a review. Curr Probl Diagn Radiol 2005;34: 106–115

Sawhney MS, Kratzke RA, Lederle FA, et al. EUS-guided FNA for the diagnosis of advanced lung cancer. Gastrointest Endosc 2006;63: 959–965

Tournoy KG, Praet MM, Van Maele G, et al. Esophageal endoscopic ultrasound with fine-needle aspiration with an on-site cytopathologist: high accuracy for the diagnosis of mediastinal lymphadenopathy. Chest 2005;128:3004–3009

Vilmann P, Krasnik M, Larsen SS, et al. Transesophageal endo-scopic ultrasound-guided fine-needle aspiration (EUS-FNA) and endo-bronchial ultrasound-guided transbronchial needle aspiration (EBUS-YBNA) biopsy: a combined approach in the evaluation of mediastinal lesions. Endoscopy 2005;37:833–839

Vincent BD, El-Bayoumi E, Hofman B, et al. Real-time endobronchial ultrasound-guided transbronchial lymph node aspiration. Ann Thorac Surg 2008;85:224–230

Yung RC. Tissue diagnosis of suspected lung cancer: selecting between bron-choscopy, transthoracic needle aspiration, and resectional biopsy. Respir Care Clin N Am 2003;9:51–76

Chapter 2
Normal Components

Epithelial Elements

Tracheal and Bronchial Respiratory Epithelium

Normal bronchial respiratory epithelium usually appears as monolayer tissue fragments and strips in bronchoscopic brush, lavage, aspirate, or transbronchial/tracheal fine needle aspirations. Epithelial cells have a uniform, honeycomb appearance *en face*, and columnar shape with basally located round uniform nuclei, terminal plates and cilia from profile (Fig. 2.1A, B & C). Rare goblet cells (Fig. 2.2) and reserve cells (Fig. 2.3) can be present; they are more frequently found in reactive conditions (see Chapter 3).

Alveolar Epithelium

Normal type 1 pneumocytes are not recognized in cytologic specimens. Type 2 pneumocytes are present in bronchoalveolar lavages (BAL) and fine needle aspirations and may resemble histiocytes, but they have denser cytoplasm and lack phagocytized material (Fig. 2.4A & B).

Non-Epithelial Cellular Elements

Specimens procured from normal individuals contain a variety of nonepithelial inflammatory cells including macrophages,

Y.S. Erozan, I. Ramzy, *Pulmonary Cytopathology*,
Essentials in Cytopathology 6, DOI 10.1007/978-0-387-88888-0_2,
© Springer Science+Business Media, LLC 2009

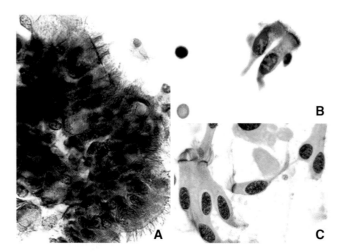

Fig. 2.1 Respiratory epithelium (**A**) A sheet of ciliated columnar cells. (**B**) Two cells with terminal bars and cilia. (**C**) The oval nuclei have finely granular open chromatin and small nucleoli (Papanicolaou, high power)

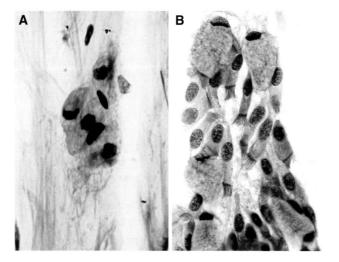

Fig. 2.2 Respiratory mucinous cells. (**A**) Columnar nonciliated cells in mucinous background, sputum. (**B**) Mucinous cells mixed with ciliated cells, bronchial brush (Papanicolaou, high power)

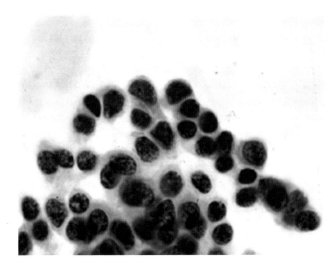

Fig. 2.3 Reserve cells with scant cyanophilic cytoplasm and small hyperchromatic nuclei. These cells are not usually encountered in bronchial material under normal conditions (Papanicolaou, oil, ×100 objective)

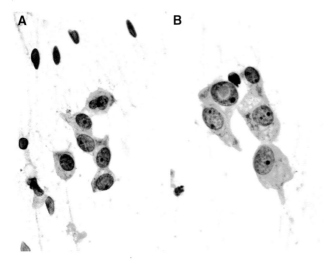

Fig. 2.4 Alveolar epithelium of type 2 pneumocytes showing in (**A**) cells with moderate amount of cytoplasm that lacks phagocytized material, unlike macrophages. (**B**) Some nuclei may have intranuclear cytoplasmic vacuoles (Papanicolaou, oil, ×100 objective)

eosinophils, neutrophils and lymphocytes. The number and type of cells is influenced by the method of sampling, processing and by presence of history of smoking. Although it is not practical to have a differential cell count, some general assessment is usually possible. Smokers, particularly those with chronic bronchitis, have larger numbers of inflammatory cells in their BAL specimens with predominance of pulmonary macrophages and neutrophils, as compared to nonsmokers. The significance of finding these cells depends on the cell type, numbers, distribution and associated lesions. They may represent reaction to injury, to a nearby neoplasm or a manifestation of a systemic process.

Macrophages and Giant Cells

These are common elements in pulmonary specimens, particularly in BAL material where they account for 60–90% of the cells (Fig. 2.5). Increased numbers of macrophages are usually

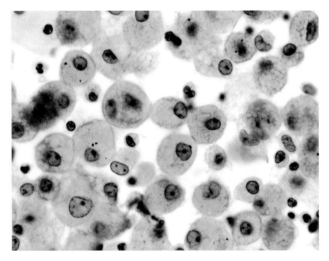

Fig. 2.5 Pulmonary macrophages with vesicular nuclei and foamy cytoplasm (Papanicolaou, oil, ×100 objective)

associated with inflammatory conditions such as pneumonia, granulomas or bronchitis. However, they can also be seen in close proximity to malignant tumors, particularly when there is extensive necrosis. The cells vary in size and have bland oval or kidney shaped nuclei with finely granular chromatin and small nucleoli. Macrophages are often multinucleated; the nuclei within each multinucleated cell are of similar size and morphology (Fig. 2.6). Rarely do these cells raise differential diagnostic challenge, in view of the evenly distributed fine chromatin and uniformly thin nuclear membrane. Reactive macrophages, however, may have large nuclei with prominent nucleoli and cytoplasmic vacuoles, raising the possibility of adenocarcinoma. The presence of a spectrum that encompasses normal and atypical macrophages with similar nuclear shapes and chromatin characteristics speaks against adenocarcinoma.

Several intrinsic and extrinsic elements can be seen within the cytoplasm of macrophages (Fig. 2.7A, B). Examples of intrinsic elements are hemosiderin, lipid, lipofuscin and blood cells. The

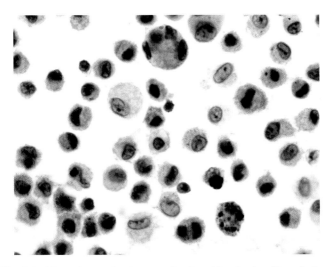

Fig. 2.6 Macrophages showing occasional multinucleation (Papanicolaou, high power)

A   B

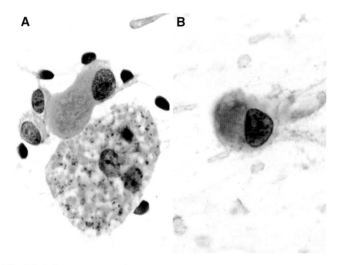

Fig. 2.7 Pulmonary macrophages with phagocytized material in (**A**). The cell in (**B**) shows dense cytoplasm and an eccentric nucleus (Papanicolaou, oil, ×100 objective)

tan brown granules seen in smokers stain positively with iron, but the granules are finer and stain less intensely than those of siderophages. Although the presence of phagocytized lipid may indicate lipid pneumonia, it can also be encountered in idiopathic pulmonary fibrosis, bronchiectasis and obstructive conditions. Extrinsic elements that may be phagocytized by macrophages include carbon particles, silica and asbestos fibers. Biologic agents such as *Mycobacterium tuberculosis* or fungi produce a reaction that often includes multinucleated giant cells and is characteristic, though not pathognomonic, of the causative organism. The histiocytic response can be altered in immunocompromised patients, as in the case of tuberculosis when Langerhan's giant cells are lacking. Identification of some organisms may be feasible on the basis of their morphology, such as in the case of coccidioidomycosis illustrated in Fig. 2.8; other organisms often require microbiologic studies of the pulmonary sample.

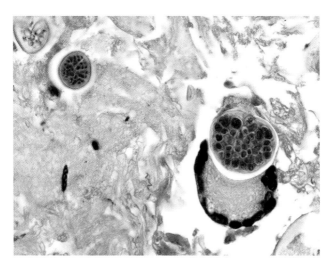

Fig. 2.8 Giant cell and necrosis. This giant cell reaction is associated with coccidioidomycosis infection (H & E, medium power)

Multinucleated giant cells, other than histiocytes, can be seen in a variety of lesions, including sarcoidosis, giant cell interstitial and viral pneumonias, especially in bronchial brushings. The cytologic features of giant cell interstitial pneumonia include large numbers of multinucleated giant cells and nonpigmented macrophages. This rare condition is associated with occupational exposure to heavy metals. Giant cells associated with viral infections are discussed later.

Siderophages

The cytoplasm of these macrophages contains golden brown hemosiderin granules that are partially refractile, unlike the dusky blue-black carbon pigment seen in anthracosis (Fig. 2.9). Siderophages are seen in patients with congestive heart failure, infarcts, and in cases of hemorrhage associated with Goodpasture syndrome, Wegener granulomatosis and idiopathic pulmonary hemosiderosis. Positive staining with Prussian blue confirms the

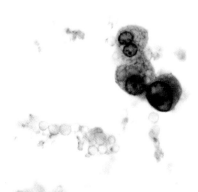

Fig. 2.9 Siderophages with opaque pigment granules that vary in size. These would stain positively with Prussian blue, and negatively with melanin immunostains, such as Melan A (Papanicolaou, oil, ×100 objective)

nature of the pigment and differentiates hemosiderin from lipofuscin and melanin.

Polymorphonuclear Leukocytes

A wide variety of conditions are associated with the presence of neutrophils in pulmonary specimens, other than contaminants from oral contents. The cells are seen in large numbers in acute bronchitis, bacterial pneumonias and abscesses. They are also encountered in BAL specimens procured from smokers, and from patients with asbestosis, idiopathic pulmonary fibrosis, scleroderma, rheumatoid arthritis, diffuse alveolar damage, adult respiratory distress syndrome and others. Acute inflammatory cell infiltrate is also frequently present as a component of the necrotic background associated with malignant neoplasms.

Lymphocytes

Small mature lymphocytes are not uncommon in specimens procured by bronchial brushings, bronchial lavage or bronchoalveolar lavage. An abundance of lymphocytes may be encountered in transbronchial Wang needle aspirates, and is an indication of adequate sampling of the hilar lymph nodes. In BAL specimens, most of the lymphocytes encountered are of T cell lineage, with a helper to suppressor ratio of 1:8. Such ratio is altered in favor of helper (CD4 positive) cells in sarcoidosis, or towards suppressor (CD8 positive) cells in hypersensitivity pneumonitis. Granulomatous and viral infections, hypersensitivity and drug-induced pneumonitis are associated with increased number of lymphocytes. In follicular bronchitis, large immature lymphocytes and tingible body macrophages are seen in addition to mature lymphocytes.

Conditions associated with abundant lymphocytes
- Granulomas (tuberculosis, sarcoidosis)
- Hypersensitivity pneumonitis
- Drug induced reactions
- Viral infections
- Lymphoma/leukemia

Differential diagnosis: Chronic inflammatory lesions may present as a mass, raising the possibility of a neoplasm. Conversely, a neoplasm may result in bronchial obstruction and subsequent chronic inflammation. In the presence of abundant lymphocytes, small cell carcinoma and lymphoma should be considered in the differential diagnosis. The nuclei of neoplastic cells of small cell carcinoma are larger than those of mature lymphocytes, with pleomorphism, molding and streaking of chromatin. Immunostains for neuroendocrine markers may be needed for differentiating the two cell types. In cases of pulmonary involvement by lymphoma or leukemia, the lymphocytic infiltrate is more prominent; adequate clinical data and submitting an aliquot for flow cytometric analysis are critical in establishing the correct diagnosis.

Eosinophils

These inflammatory cells account only for 1% of cells in BAL material in normal individuals. They are usually seen in response to antigenic stimulation, such as in bronchial asthma, parasitic and fungal infections, hypersensitivity pneumonitis and in eosinophilic pneumonia. On Papanicolaou stained material, eosinophils do not exhibit the bright red or pink granules seen with Romanowsky stains; instead, the granules are somewhat yellowish green and refractile, and the cells are easily recognized by their characteristic bilobed nuclei (Fig. 2.10). Abundant eosinophils are associated with rhomboid Charcot–Leyden crystals, which are described later.

Conditions associated with abundant eosinophils

- Hypersensitivity pneumonitis
- Drug induced reactions
- Parasitic infestations
- Bronchial asthma
- Eosinophilic pneumonia

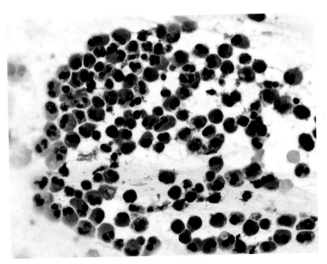

Fig. 2.10 Eosinophils in large numbers in sputum from a patient with allergic pneumonitis of undetermined etiology (Papanicolaou, medium power)

Megakaryocytes

Though often seen in alveolar septa, megakaryocytes are rarely encountered in respiratory cytologic specimens. They are characterized by multiple nuclei that are centrally located. The nuclei are hyperchromatic and pleomorphic, unlike the uniform vesicular nuclei of histiocytic giant cells.

Miscellaneous Noncellular Elements

Curschmann Spirals

These are mucous casts of medium-sized to small bronchioles that are commonly found in sputa of heavy smokers. They can also be encountered in material procured from patients with bronchial asthma, chronic bronchitis and other obstructive lung disease. They form corkscrew like spirals, each has a central core from which filamentous structures radiate perpendicular to the longitudinal axis of the core. Curschmann spirals stain pale cyanophilic or eosinophilic with Papanicolaou and black with silver stains (Fig. 2.11A,B).

Charcot–Leyden Crystals

These crystals form as a result of condensation of the cytoplasmic granules of eosinophils. These are rhomboidal or needle-shaped structures of variable sizes and stain green or red on Papanicolaou stained material, with sharply defined and refractile edges (Fig. 2.12). Charcot–Leyden crystals can be observed in many conditions in which there is increased number of eosinophils, such as in bronchial asthma or allergic pneumonitis due to different causes.

Blue Bodies (Corpora amylacea)

Corpora amylacea are globular structures that form within alveolar spaces, and are more likely to be associated with pulmonary

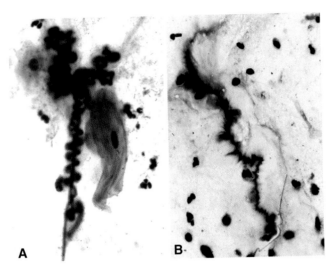

Fig. 2.11 Curschmann spiral. The inspissated mucus is a cast of bronchial lumen (**A** & **B** Papanicolaou and Diff-Quik , medium power). Reproduced from Ostrowski MO and Ramzy I, *In: Ramzy I: Clinical Cytopathology and Aspiration Biopsy, ed 2, New York, NY, McGraw-Hill, 2001,* with permission of The McGraw-Hill Companies

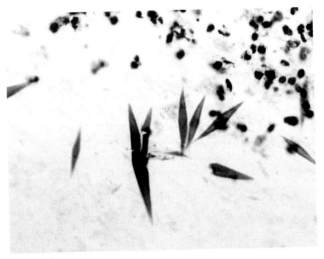

Fig. 2.12 Charcot–Leyden crystals. Sputum from a patient with bronchial asthma. The rhomboid crystals vary in size and stain greenish or red with Papanicolaou stain (Papanicolaou, medium power)

edema, infarction or chronic bronchitis. The acellular bodies are large and spherical, with a central birefringent core that is surrounded by homogeneous or lamellated material (Fig. 2.13). Although concentric laminations may be seen, they do not calcify similar to psammoma bodies. Identification of corpora amylacea has no clinical significance.

Calcific and Psammoma Bodies

Calcified irregularly shaped structures can be encountered in chronic granulomas, such as tuberculosis, and are nonspecific. Well organized lamellated calcified psammoma bodies may be seen in a variety of primary or metastatic papillary neoplasms. These include bronchioloalveolar carcinoma, metastatic thyroid carcinoma and ovarian carcinoma (Fig. 2.14A, B). The presence of psammoma bodies should not be taken as conclusive evidence

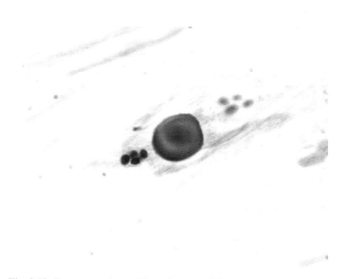

Fig. 2.13 Corpora amylacea. The pale cyanophilic structures may show faint lamination but are not calcified (Papanicolaou, high power)

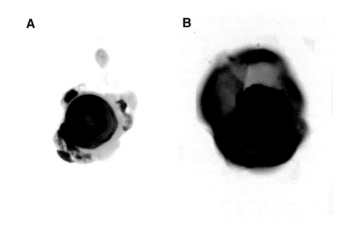

Fig. 2.14 Psammoma bodies. (**A** and **B**) The lamellated calcified structures can be encountered in benign and malignant lesions (Papanicolaou, high power)

of malignancy in the absence of epithelial cells with clear nuclear features of malignancy. Other lesions, including the rare benign condition of alveolar microlithiasis, may be associated with psammoma bodies.

Contaminants

A wide variety of food particles, such as vegetable material and meat fibers, as well as bacterial colonies, pollen and other debris may be encountered in specimens arriving to the laboratory (Fig. 2.15A, B). Some of these may superficially resemble fungal organisms or even squamous cells, but establishing their nature as oral contaminants does not present a problem in most cases (Fig. 2.16). The significance of finding bacteria or fungi may not be clear in some cases, and clinical correlation as well as radiologic correlation are necessary. Presence of food particles is rarely an indication of pulmonary aspiration.

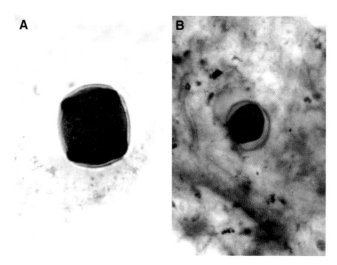

Fig. 2.15 Plant cells. (**A**) Pollens and (**B**) Plant cells. Note characteristic refractile cell walls and often geometric patterns that easily distinguish these from keratinized squamous cells (Papanicolaou, high power)

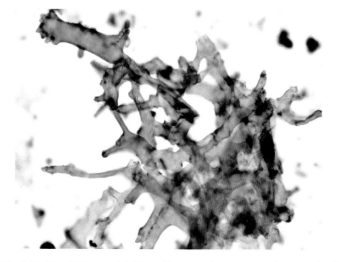

Fig. 2.16 Vegetable material. These fibers may be encountered as a result of oral contamination of the specimen. Their irregular diameters help differentiating them from zygomycetes (Papanicolaou, medium power)

Suggested Reading

Antonakopoulos GN, Lambrinaki E, Kyrkou KA. Curschmann's spirals in sputum: histochemical evidence of bronchial gland ductal origin. Diagn Cytopathol 1987;3:291–294

Chen KTK. Psammoma bodies in fine-needle aspiration cytology of papillary adenocarcinoma of the lung. Diagn Cytopathol 1990;6:235–242

Chapter 3
Hyperplasia, Reactive Changes and Metaplasia

The epithelium of the respiratory tract responds to injury in several ways that include hyperplasia, metaplasia, degeneration, repair, inflammation or neoplasia. Although these are often non-specific reactions, others have characteristic cytologic features that point to specific etiology. Recognizing these reactive changes as manifested in cytologic specimens is critical, particularly since some may be misinterpreted as neoplastic transformation of the epithelium.

Hyperplastic and Reactive Changes

Goblet Cell Hyperplasia

Goblet cells are mucinous cells that are present between ciliated columnar cells lining the bronchi, gradually decreasing in number as they approach the terminal bronchioles. Their proliferation is often one of the early responses to various irritants, including allergens, environmental toxins, or smoke. Goblet cell hyperplasia is also a major component of the response to chronic inflammation, chronic bronchitis, or bronchiectasis. These cells also proliferate in association with bronchial asthma. In cytologic material, the cells often appear as clusters, particularly in bronchial brushings, or singly. The individual cells have a hyperdistended mucinous vacuole or multiple smaller vacuoles that distend the cell.

Y.S. Erozan, I. Ramzy, *Pulmonary Cytopathology*,
Essentials in Cytopathology 6, DOI 10.1007/978-0-387-88888-0_3,
© Springer Science+Business Media, LLC 2009

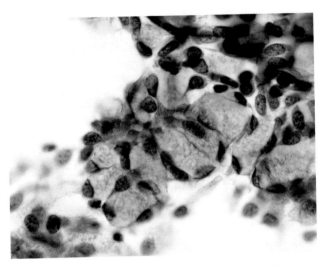

Fig. 3.1 Goblet cell metaplasia. Distention of the cytoplasm by mucinous material, pushing the nucleus to the cell base. The nuclei are uniform, unlike those of adenocarcinoma (Papanicolaou, high power)

The flattened nuclei are basally located against the cell membrane (Fig. 3.1).

Differential diagnosis: Mucinous carcinoma shows abundance of isolated cells rather than sheets, and lacks the intimate association of the mucinous cells with normal ciliated columnar cells. In addition, malignant nuclear features such as hyperchromasia, membrane irregularities and chromatin clumping are evident in carcinoma.

Reactive and Hyperplastic Bronchial Epithelium

Reactive and reparative changes are frequent cytologic findings, often associated with hyperplasia of the bronchial epithelium. They occur in response to a wide variety of conditions including pneumonia, bronchitis, bronchiectasis, bronchial asthma, and exposure to toxins, radiation, or chemotherapeutic agents. Viral pneumonias are frequently associated with prominent hyperplasia of the bronchial and alveolar epithelia. Reactive changes may

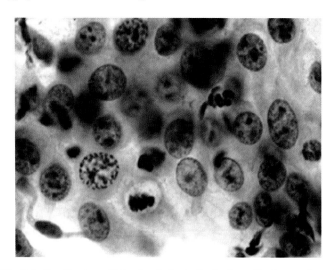

Fig. 3.2 Reactive bronchial cells. A sheet of cohesive cells shows enlarged but normochromic nuclei and prominent nucleoli. Note degenerative changes in the form of karyorrhexis. Occasional mitotic figures may be present (Papanicolaou, oil, ×100 objective). Reproduced from Ostrowski MO and Ramzy I, *In: Ramzy I: Clinical Cytopathology and Aspiration Biopsy, ed 2, New York, NY, McGraw-Hill, 2001,* with permission of The McGraw-Hill Companies

also be encountered as a result of instrumentation such as following bronchoscopy. Reactive cells usually form sheets with poorly defined individual cell borders. They have enlarged oval to round nuclei that show some variation in nuclear size (Fig. 3.2). The chromatin is usually bland, finely granular and evenly distributed throughout the nucleus. Occasional prominent chromocenters may be present. A characteristic feature is the presence of prominent nucleoli, compared to those of resting columnar cells. These nucleoli remain uniform in size and shape. Several mitotic figures may be encountered as a manifestation of the reparative or reactive process (Fig. 3.3). Multinucleated columnar cells are often present, particularly as a result of irritation caused by instrumentation and brushings, and such cells possess oval nuclei that are uniform in size with a thin nuclear membrane and small nucleoli. The lack of any significant nuclear atypia and the identification of an occasional terminal bar or cilia in nearby cells with similar nuclei help to recognize these multinucleated cells as benign bronchial cells.

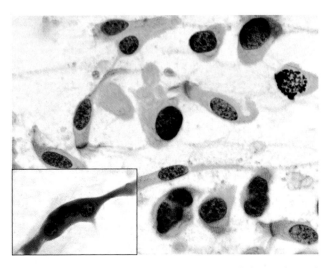

Fig. 3.3 Reactive bronchial cells. Note nuclear size variation and hyperchromasia. *Inset* depicts a multinucleated columnar cell; such appearance may be the result of disappearance of membranes separating several degenerating cells (Papanicolaou, high power)

Key features
- Cohesive cellular sheets
- Large nuclei with slight variation in size
- Chromatin evenly distributed
- Prominent nucleoli, uniform in size and shape
- Preserved terminal bars or cilia
- Multinucleation

Differential diagnosis: Adenocarcinoma, and to a lesser extent squamous cell carcinoma, share several features with reactive cells. This creates diagnostic difficulties, particularly when the reparative changes are extensive rather than focal, resulting in the presence of large numbers of atypical cells. Reactive cells are unlikely to be associated with necrotic tumor diatheses, clustering and syncytia-like formations with nuclear overlapping characteristic of malignant cells. Although the nuclei of reactive cells may vary in size, such variation is not as prominent as that observed in malignant cells (see Fig. 7.22 for comparison). The nuclear membranes are generally smooth and regular, and the nuclei lack the irregular chromatin clumping and irregular nucleoli of adenocarcinoma cells. The presence of a continuum that bridges the gap between normal looking columnar cells and atypical ones supports a benign diagnosis. In exceptionally difficult cases when the cells show indeterminate features, a repeat cytologic examination or procuring material by a different sampling technique may help in correctly identifying the exact underlying process. In our experience, open lines of communication between the radiologist, pulmonologist and cytopathologist play a major role in solving these problem cases and ensuring optimal care for the patient.

Reactive Terminal Bronchial/Alveolar Epithelium

The peripheral parts of the lung, comprising alveoli and associated smaller branches of the bronchial tree, react to injuries in a different way from the epithelium lining the main bronchi. Sampling of the peripheral areas is possible usually through bronchoalveolar lavage (BAL) and through needle aspiration biopsy. The epithelial cells procured from terminal bronchioles or alveoli are usually smaller than those obtained from the main bronchi. They also form smaller clusters with fewer cells each; many appear as isolated cells. These small cells often show marked nuclear enlargement and atypia (Fig. 3.4). Proliferation of alveolar macrophages and type II pneumocytes can be induced by several conditions, including viral pneumonias, interstitial lung disease, and infarction, organizing pneumonia, asbestosis and some drug-mediated changes (Fig. 3.5). The proliferation of type II pneumocytes can be pronounced in the case of viral pneumonia associated with diffuse alveolar damage. The majority of the cells, particularly macrophages, appear isolated. However, proliferating type II pneumocytes may form papillary clusters with cytoplasmic vacuoles, simulating well differentiated adenocarcinoma of the acinar, papillary or bronchioloalveolar type.

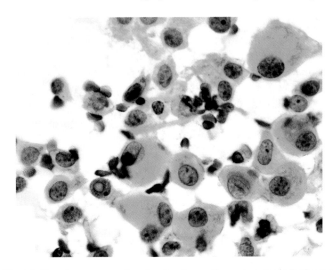

Fig. 3.4 Reactive pneumocytes. An abundance of pneumocytes in BAL specimen; some nuclei show intranuclear vacuoles (Papanicolaou, high power)

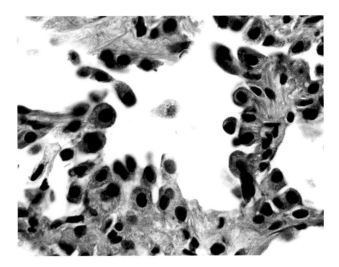

Fig. 3.5 Reactive pneumocytes. FNA specimen from a patient with Nocardia infection. Note the similarity of the histologic features to those of bronchioloalveolar carcinoma illustrated in Fig. 7.27 (Cell block, H & E, high power)

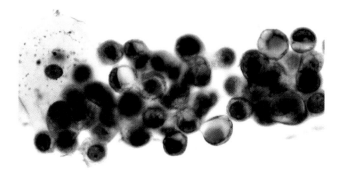

Fig. 3.6 Atypical bronchial cells. Note nuclear hyperchromasia and size variation in this material, procured from a 91-year-old man with a long history of smoking. Careful examination may reveal some cilia, thus supporting the benign nature of such cells (Papanicolaou, high power)

Key features
- Clusters smaller than bronchial reactive cells
- Cells smaller and fewer per cluster
- Type II pneumocytes with papillary formations
- Marked nuclear enlargement
- Abundant isolated macrophages

Differential diagnosis: Well differentiated adenocarcinoma cells possess more hyperchromatic nuclei with thick nuclear membrane and often display intranuclear inclusions, unlike reactive epithelial cells (see Fig. 7.22 and Table 7.3). It is important to recognize that foci of type II pneumocyte hyperplasia may be encountered adjacent to bronchioloalveolar carcinoma. Distinguishing reactive terminal bronchioloalveolar epithelium from carcinoma is occasionally very difficult, and the clinician, radiologist and cytopathologist may have to resort to repeat sampling or open biopsy if suspicion of malignancy lingers in their minds (Fig. 3.6).

Reserve Cell Hyperplasia

Bronchial reserve cells are small round to polygonal cells located in the mucosa close to the basement membrane, between the basal parts of ciliated columnar cells. These are multipotent cells that increase in number in response to several factors, particularly exposure to smoke and other chemical irritants. They are seen in specimens procured by brushing or washing of large bronchi, forming small cohesive clusters or tissue fragments rather than isolated cells. Their cyanophilic cytoplasm is scant and surrounds small round to slightly oval nuclei that have bland uniformly distributed chromatin (Fig. 3.7). A few ciliated bronchial cells, with more abundant cytoplasm, as well as some metaplastic squamous cells may be observed around the rim of some of the larger tissue fragments.

Key features
- Small groups or fragments
- Scant cyanophilic cytoplasm
- Small oval nuclei with bland chromatin
- Association with a few ciliated columnar cells

Differential diagnosis: Small cell carcinoma is the most critical differential diagnostic problem. The number of tissue fragments

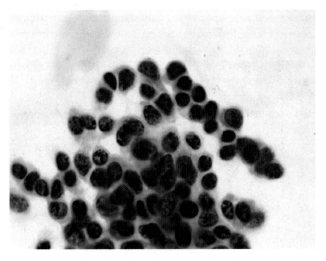

Fig. 3.7 Reserve cell hyperplasia. Abundant small cells with scant cytoplasm appearing as sheets or isolated cells (Papanicolaou, high power)

and isolated cells is usually greater in small cell carcinoma, with necrotic material in the background. The nuclei of small cell carcinoma are pleomorphic, hyperchromatic, often naked, and show molding. Imaging studies usually reveal a mass in the case of carcinoma (Figs. 7.42 and 7.43, Table 7.4). Cell cohesion observed in reserve cell hyperplasia differentiates it from lymphoma/leukemia.

Ciliocytophthoria

First reported by Papanicolaou, ciliocytophthoria was thought to be specific for viral infections, particularly those caused by adenovirus. It is now recognized that several other reactive and degenerative conditions that affect ciliated cells can produce ciliocytophthoria. The degenerating cell is often eosinophilic, and gradually develops a narrowing in the middle, with eventual separation of the cell into two parts. The basal part surrounds a small pyknotic nucleus, while the apical part has the remainder of the cytoplasm with the attached ciliary tuft (Fig. 3.8).

Differential diagnosis: Squamous cell carcinoma may exfoliate individual keratinized cells that are eosinophilic and possess pyknotic nuclei. However, usually more than one cell is encountered and their nuclei are irregular, unlike ciliocytophthoria where only a rare cell with a small dark but uniform nucleus is encountered.

Creola Bodies

Patients with chronic bronchitis, particularly due to asthma, frequently exfoliate papillary fragments or sheets of reactive bronchial cells that may resemble adenocarcinoma (Fig. 3.9). The fragments are also often seen in other reactive or inflammatory lesions of the bronchial mucosa. The clusters of bronchial mucosa are partially covered by ciliated respiratory epithelium. Because of the thickness of the tissue fragment, accurate visualization of detail of the crowded nuclei is difficult. When visualized around the edge of the fragment, the nuclei are bland with evenly distributed chromatin, smooth nuclear outline and uniform nuclear membrane. Small nucleoli may be present. Identification of cilia

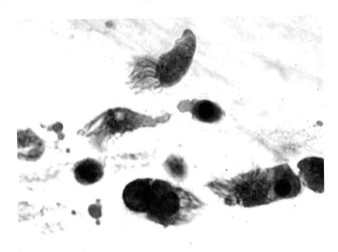

Fig. 3.8 Ciliocytophthoria. There is separation of the ciliary tuft and apical cytoplasm from the nucleus in the basal part. Such degenerative change is not limited to viral infections as previously thought (Papanicolaou, oil, ×100 objective). Reproduced from Ostrowski MO and Ramzy I, *In: Ramzy I: Clinical Cytopathology and Aspiration Biopsy, ed 2, New York, NY, McGraw-Hill, 2001,* with permission of The McGraw-Hill Companies

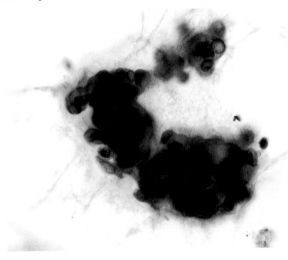

Fig. 3.9 Creola body. The cluster of respiratory cells may show hyperchromatic nuclei, but careful examination reveals cilia or terminal bars at the edge of some cells, supporting their benign nature (Papanicolaou, high power)

lined up along the edge of the cluster is reassuring and can be facilitated by partial closure of the microscope's condenser.

Key features
- Sheets or thick 3-D tissue fragments
- Cell borders poorly defined
- Crowded but uniform bland nuclei
- Small nucleoli
- Cilia or terminal bars at edge or middle

Differential diagnosis: Adenocarcinoma shows more isolated cells, with nuclear features of malignancy such as pleomorphism and hyperchromasia. Examination of the epithelial sheets and clusters fails to demonstrate cilia in malignant cells.

Squamous Metaplasia and Atypia

Squamous metaplasia is a common mechanism by which the columnar respiratory epithelium reacts to sustained injury resulting from exposure to chemical, physical or biologic agents. The most common of these agents are cigarette smoke and chronic infections, particularly organizing pneumonia, usual interstitial pneumonia (UIP), and fungal infections. Dr. Papanicolaou described small eosinophilic "Pap cells" in his own sputum; they turned out to be the result of an infection. Ischemic changes due to pulmonary infarction and long standing granulomatous infections, such as tuberculosis and chronic lung abscesses, can also induce squamous metaplasia. The oval or elliptical cells appear as small miniature keratinized squamous cells with bright orangeophilic or cyanophilic cytoplasm (Fig. 3.10A, B, C). Their nuclei are pyknotic small and uniform. Nuclear atypia, however, may be prominent particularly in cells derived from long standing abscesses, organizing pneumonias or tuberculous cavities (Fig. 3.11A, B). Bronchial squamous metaplasia with atypia may also precede dysplastic change and the subsequent development of squamous cell carcinoma in some cases; hence they should be noted in the cytopathology report for further monitoring of the patient (see Chap. 7).

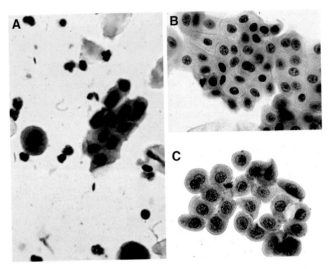

Fig. 3.10 Squamous metaplasia (**A**, **B** and **C**). These cells are common in sputa from smokers. The cells are often smaller than normal squames derived from the oral cavity, and the cytoplasm can be orangeophilic, brown or cyanophilic (Papanicolaou, **A** & **B** medium power, **C** high power)

Key features

- Oval or elliptical small cells (miniature squames)
- Bright orangeophilic cytoplasm
- Nuclei pyknotic, small and uniform
- Marked nuclear atypia should raise concern

Differential diagnosis: Keratinizing squamous cell carcinoma can be difficult to differentiate from atypical squamous metaplasia. The diagnosis can be problematic for treating physicians, radiologists and pathologists alike, since both conditions can be associated with cavitary lesions or central necrosis, and only a few cells are encountered in exfoliated material. Needle aspiration biopsy specimens, however, present less of a challenge; the presence of large numbers of atypical cells, particularly if their nuclei are pleomorphic, supports the diagnosis of malignancy. Since nuclear atypia in metaplastic cells may be a reflection of a squamous metaplasia-dysplasia-carcinoma spectrum, both conditions may coexist.

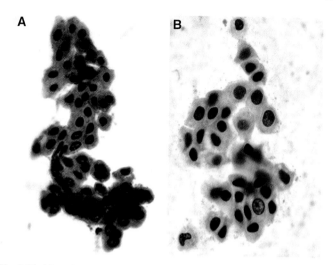

Fig. 3.11 Metaplastic and atypical squamous cells. (**A** & **B**) Sheets of squamous cells from an aspirate of a right lung mass. Some cells showing nuclear hyperchromasia. These may be a marker for subsequent or concomitant development of squamous cancer. However, in this case, they were derived from the wall of a chronic abscess cavity (Papanicolaou, high power)

Therapy-Induced Changes

Radiation Therapy

The lung may be exposed to radiation during treatment of primary and metastatic neoplasms such as breast cancer. The effects mostly involve the respiratory epithelium, and include nuclear and cytoplasmic changes which are shared by squamous and columnar cells. There is cytomegaly due to enlargement of both the nucleus and cytoplasm, thus the N/C ratio is generally preserved (Fig. 3.12). Many bizarre shaped cells are encountered and several of these may be multinucleated. Nuclear chromatin is smudged or shows coarse clumping, and degenerative vacuoles may be seen within the nucleus. The cytoplasm is often cloudy and exhibits debris and vacuoles of variable sizes. Dual staining of the cytoplasm, with cyanophilic and eosinophilic areas may be seen. The glandular cells maintain their columnar shapes, and remnants

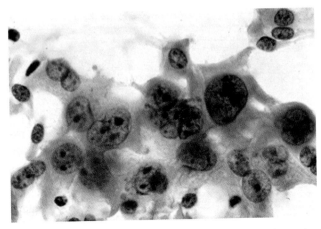

Fig. 3.12 Radiation effects. Marked concomitant nuclear and cytoplasmic enlargement, with normal N/C ratio. Degenerative changes, such as nuclear and cytoplasmic vacuoles, multinucleation, bizarre shapes and cloudy cytoplasm are also encountered (Papanicolaou, oil, ×100 objective). Reproduced from Ostrowski MO and Ramzy I, *In: Ramzy I: Clinical Cytopathology and Aspiration Biopsy, ed 2, New York, NY, McGraw-Hill, 2001,* with permission of The McGraw-Hill Companies

of cilia or terminal bars may still be identified. Various inflammatory cells, including histiocytes, may be seen in response to the physical injury and the repair process that follows. In some cases, squamous metaplasia of the columnar epithelium is noted and may be associated with atypical nuclei.

Key features
- Cytomegaly and karyomegaly with preservation of N/C ratio
- Bizarre-shaped cells
- Nuclei with smudged chromatin
- Degenerative nuclear vacuoles
- Cloudy cytoplasm with debris and vacuoles
- Amphophilic staining of cytoplasm
- Multinucleation

Differential diagnosis: Coagulative necrosis of respiratory columnar cells may give the impression of squamous cell carcinoma. The preservation of N/C ratio and the degenerative nuclear and cytoplasmic changes help in distinguishing radiation effect from carcinoma. With the availability of history of a previously treated malignancy, the diagnosis of radiation injury does not present a problem in most cases. However, distinction between radiation effects and recurrent or resistant tumor cells can be problematic. A definitive diagnosis of malignancy requires identification of well preserved cells with sharply defined nuclear membranes, crisp chromatin and no evidence of degenerative changes in the cytoplasm. The cytologic features of the material should also be compared and correlated to any previous samples from the tumor.

Chemotherapy

The effects of chemotherapeutic drugs are not specific, and usually most prominent in alveolar pneumocytes and the respiratory columnar epithelium procured by BAL. In the majority of cases, only a few cells encountered will show the cytologic changes of chemotherapy. The columnar cells show features similar to those encountered following radiotherapy, with cytomegaly, karyomegaly, macronucleoli and preservation of N/C ratio. Degenerative changes in both the nucleus and cytoplasm and bizarre shaped cells are also seen with the use of chemotherapeutic agents. The cells may maintain their cilia in the process, further supporting their benign nature (Figs. 3.13 and 3.14A). Some drugs, such as Busulfan, can induce marked interstitial fibrosis, while others may cause prominent alveolar hyperplasia or eosinophilia. Bleomycin is associated with squamous cell atypia but does not manifest changes in columnar cells, while BCNU is associated with giant cells and changes that may resemble adenocarcinoma.

Key features
- Mostly in alveolar pneumocytes and columnar cells
- Similar to radiation changes
- Prominent alveolar hyperplasia
- Squamous cell atypia with Bleomycin
- Giant cells with BCNU

Differential diagnosis: The changes induced by chemotherapy are not specific and should be differentiated from those of other

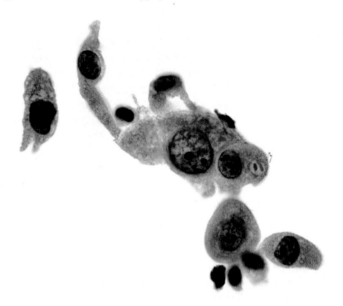

Fig. 3.13 Chemotherapeutic changes in BAL, in a patient receiving therapy for late stage colon cancer. The cytoplasm and nuclei of individual cells show concomitant enlargement and nuclear detail is blurred (Papanicolaou, oil, ×100 objective). Slide courtesy of Dr. Barbara Steel, Middletown, OH

drugs that can affect respiratory and bronchioloalveolar epithelia. Careful inquiry about the history and time of administering the drug is critical in these cases. Chemotherapeutic effects should also be differentiated from viable or recurrent tumor. Presence of only a few isolated cells, rather than sheets or large clusters, smudging of nuclear chromatin and cytoplasmic degenerative changes favor the diagnosis of chemotherapy effect.

Nonchemotherapeutic Drugs

Nitrofurantoin and sulfasalazine may induce eosinophilic pneumonia, interstitial inflammation or diffuse alveolar damage. The resulting changes are not reflected in a characteristic cytomorpho-

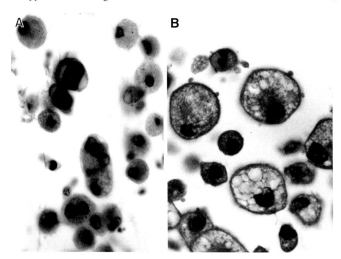

Fig. 3.14 Iatrogenic atypical respiratory cells. (**A**) Cytologic atypia in a bronchial lavage material procured from an immunosuppressed patient post bone marrow transplant. Note presence of cilia in the cells depicting enlarged nuclei (Papanicolaou, high power). (**B**) Amiodarone effects result in multiple cytoplasmic vacuoles that occupy most of the cytoplasm (Diff-Quik, Oil, X100 Objective). Slide from Ostrowski MO, Ramzy I, *In Ramzy I*: Clinical Cytopathology and Aspiration biopsy, ed 2, New York, McGraw-Hill, 2000, with permission

logic pattern. The antiarrhythmic drug amiodarone can also cause pulmonary reaction, usually in the form of alveolitis, bronchiolitis obliterans organizing pneumonia (BOOP) or pleural effusion. Cytologic material procured from patients receiving amiodarone shows characteristic vacuolated foam cells. The cytoplasmic vacuoles are uniform, poorly-defined and smaller than those seen in lipid pneumonia. They are also oil red O negative (Fig. 3.14 B).

Pulmonary Allograft Transplants

The four years survival rate for recipients of pulmonary allografts has increased to around 50%, and these patients continue to be at risk of rejection and infection. Rejection may be acute, chronic bronchial or chronic vascular, and may be associated with lymphocytic bronchitis or bronchiolitis. Examination of cytologic material does not play a significant role in the assessment or grading of rejection, since these require bronchoscopic biopsies. Cytologic studies, however, can help in management, since these patients are also highly susceptible to infections. Some infections, such as Gram-negative bacilli and coagulase-positive staphylococci, require microbiologic studies for identification, while others have fairly characteristic cytomorphologic features. Examples of the latter group include Cytomegalovirus, Candida spp., Aspergillus spp. and *Pneumocystis jiroveci* as discussed below under "Infections."

Pneumoconioses

Although the original definition of these non-neoplastic lesions was limited to those caused by industrial exposure to mineral dust, it has been recently expanded to encompass inorganic and organic particles, chemical fumes and vapors.

Asbestosis

Exposure to asbestos is very common, particularly in workers in insulation, fire retardant, shipyard, brake, mining and cement industries. Prolonged exposure, particularly when combined with smoking, may induce asbestosis after a long latent period, resulting in interstitial pulmonary fibrosis and pleural plaques. The needle shaped clear fibers are 5–200 µm long, 2–5 µm wide and by themselves are almost invisible on Papanicolaou stain. Identification in cytologic specimens, however, is facilitated by the encasement of the central fiber by an iron-positive golden brown refractile proteinaceous coat that is often segmented, with bulbous "dumbbell-like" swelling at each end (Fig. 3.15A, B). These bodies are also referred to as "ferruginous bodies," although that term includes other mineral fibers coated by glycoproteins and hemosiderin, such as the black fibers of titanium oxide. BAL

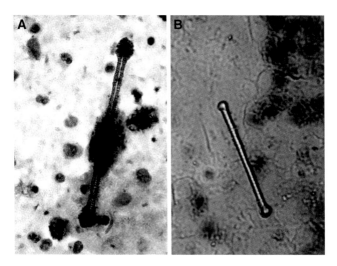

Fig. 3.15 Asbestosis. (**A**) A ferruginous body in sputum showing segmented encrustation surrounding the fiber. (**B**) A yellowish brown refractile structure with a bulbous swelling at each end (Papanicolaou, medium power)

material tends to be more sensitive to detection of asbestos bodies in patients with lung disease than sputum examination (75% vs 25%). The identification of large numbers of asbestos bodies in pulmonary cytologic material of any source is a significant finding, but their presence in small numbers is nonspecific as an indicator for industrial exposure. In addition to interstitial fibrosis, asbestosis is often associated with squamous metaplasia, dysplasia or malignancy. Asbestosis patients who are also smokers have a 30–40% risk of developing lung cancer, and careful search for early epithelial changes in cytologic specimens is critical.

Key features
- Needle-shaped clear fibers
- Refractile golden brown segmented proteinaceous coat
- Coat is iron-positive (ferruginous body)
- Macrophages may surround or engulf some fibers

Other Pneumoconioses

Carbon, silica, beryllium, zirconium, iron oxide, cotton, moldy hay and many air pollutants can induce a spectrum of lesions that encompasses fibrosis, allergic response, acute respiratory distress syndrome, granulomas, neoplasms of lung and pleura, among others. A detailed discussion of these pneumoconioses is beyond the scope of this volume; they do not present specific features that allow identification of the causative agent in cytologic material, with rare exceptions such as beryllium or zirconium granulomas.

Suggested Reading

Aisner SC, Gupta PK, Frost JK. Sputum cytology in pulmonary sarcoidosis. Acta Cytol 1997;21:394–398

Akoun GM, Gauther-Rahaman S, Milleron BJ, et al. Amiodarone-induced hypersensitivity pneumonitis. Chest 1984;85:133–135

Angeles R, Gong Y. Fine-needle aspiration cytology of a rheumatoid arthritis-associated interstitial lung disease. Diagn Cytopathol. 2008;36:686–688

Bedrossian CWM, Corey BJ. Abnormal sputum cytopathology during chemotherapy with bleomycin. Acta Cytol 1978;22:202–207

Cordeiro CR, Jones JC, Alfaro T, Ferreira AJ. Bronchoalveolar lavage in occupational lung diseases. Semin Respir Crit Care Med. 2007:504–513. Review

Frost JK, Gupta PK, Erozan YS. Pulmonary cytologic observation in toxic environment inhalations. Hum Pathol 1973;4:521–526

Grotte D, Stanley MW, Swanson PE, et al. Reactive type II pneumocytes in bronchoalveolar lavage fluid from adult respiratory distress syndrome can be mistaken for cells of adenocarcinoma. Diagn Cytopathol 1990;6: 317–322

Martin WJ, Osborn MJ, Douglas WW. Amiodarone pulmonary toxicity: assessments, bronchoalveolar lavage. Chest 1985;88:630–631

Monabati A, Ghayumi MA, Kumar P. Familial pulmonary alveolar microlithiasis diagnosed by bronchoalveolar lavage. A case report. Acta Cytol 2007;51:80–82

Naryshkin S, Young NA. Respiratory cytology: a review of non-neoplastic mimics of malignancy. Diagn Cytopathol 1993;9:89–97

Naylor B, Railey C. A pitfall in the cytodiagnosis of sputum of asthmatics. J Clin Pathol 1964;17:84–89

Oztek I, Baloglu H, Uskent N, et al. Chemotherapy- and radiotherapy-induced cytologic alterations in the sputum of patients with inoperable lung carcinoma. Acta Cytol 1996;40:1265–1271

Papanicolaou GN. Degenerative changes in ciliated cells exfoliating from the bronchial epithelium as a cytologic criterion in the diagnosis of diseases of the lung. NY State J Med 1956;56:2647–2650

Ramzy I, Geraghty R, Lefcoe MS, et al. Chronic eosinophilic pneumonia: diagnosis by fine needle aspiration. Acta Cytol 1978;22:366–369

Roggli VL, Piantadosi CA, Bell DY. Asbestos bodies in bronchoalveolar lavage fluid. A study of 20 asbestos-exposed individuals and comparison to patients with other chronic interstitial lung disease. Acta Cytol 1986;30:470–476

Roggli VL, Coin PG, MacIntyre NR, et al. Asbestos content of bronchoalveolar lavage fluid: a comparison of light and scanning electron microscopic analysis. Acta Cytol 1994;38:502–510

Saito Y, Imai T, Sato M, et al. Cytologic study of tissue repair in human bronchial epithelium. Acta Cytol 1988;32:622–628

Scoggins WG, Smith RH, Frable WJ, et al. False positive cytologic diagnosis of lung carcinoma in patients with pulmonary infarcts. Ann Thorac Surg 1977;24:474–480

Selvaggi SM. Bronchoalveolar lavage in lung transplant patients. Acta Cytol 1992;36:674–679

Setta JH, Neder JA, Bagatin E, et al. Relationship between induced sputum cytology and inflammatory status with lung structural and functional abnormalities in asbestosis. Am J Ind Med. 2008 Mar;51(3):186–194

Swank PR, Greenberg SD, Hunter NR, et al. Identification of features of metaplastic cells in sputum for the detection of squamous-cell carcinoma of the lung. Diagn Cytopathol 1989;5:98–103

Chapter 4
Respiratory Infections

The wide spectrum of biologic agents to which the lung may be exposed induces different responses in the lining epithelium and surrounding tissues. The resulting cytologic alterations can be specific in some cases, while in other circumstances the reaction may be nonspecific. A granulomatous response, as an example, can be induced by bacteria, fungi, spirochetes, or parasites. However, it can also be in response to drugs, chemicals, hypersensitivity or to the presence of a neoplasm. Granulomas can present as coin lesions with clinical and imaging features that overlap with tumors. The use of BAL has reduced the need for open biopsy to investigate infectious disease in many cases. Special stains, immunostains and microbiologic cultures can be very helpful in correctly identifying the underlying pathogenetic mechanism. The discussion that follows considers viral, bacterial, mycotic and parasitic infections that have fairly characteristic cytomorphologic features.

Viral Infections

Some of the most common forms of infections encountered in the upper and lower respiratory tracts are caused by viruses. A few viruses, such as cytomegalovirus, produce fairly specific cytologic changes, while others have features that are shared by other viruses or are nonspecific. Identification of a specific virus often requires

Y.S. Erozan, I. Ramzy, *Pulmonary Cytopathology*,
Essentials in Cytopathology 6, DOI 10.1007/978-0-387-88888-0_4,
© Springer Science+Business Media, LLC 2009

immunocytochemistry, culture, DNA in situ hybridization or polymerase chain reaction (PCR). Detection of changes characteristic of one infection does not negate the need to look for features of others, particularly in immunocompromised patients who are highly susceptible to multiple infections.

Herpes Simplex Infection

Herpetic infections are often encountered in conditions associated with immunosuppression, such as in patients suffering of AIDS, undergoing chemotherapy, immunotherapy, transplant surgery or having systemic debilitating diseases such as diabetes. The cytologic features of this necrotizing type of pneumonia can be subtle. In sputum or lavage specimens, the changes are usually detected in strips of epithelium and in isolated cells within a necrotic background and acute inflammatory exudate. The characteristic cells are large and result from fusion of several cells, with multiple molded nuclei filling the entire cytoplasmic mass. The nuclear chromatin is bland and may have a relatively clear gelatinous appearance, with condensation against the inner surface of the nuclear envelop (Cowdry type 1 inclusion). In other nuclei, the inclusion forms a single well defined central structure, surrounded by a halo that separates it from the peripheral condensed chromatin (Cowdry type 2 inclusion). Both types of intranuclear inclusions represent various stages of viral effects, rather than an indication of a primary vs a secondary infection as previously suggested (Figs. 4.1 and 4.2).

Key Features
- Strips and isolated cells with cytopathic changes
- Few diagnostic multinucleated cells
- Nuclei mold and occupy most of the cell
- Single, well-defined nuclear inclusions with a halo or bland gelatinous appearing chromatin with condensation against the nuclear envelope
- Peripheral chromatin condensation
- Necrotic background with acute inflammatory cells

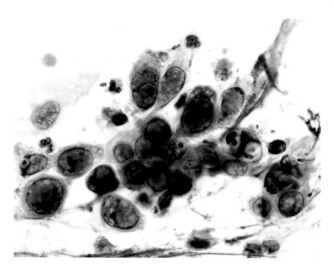

Fig. 4.1 *Herpes simplex*. The multiple nuclei occupy the entire cell, with molding and peripheral condensation of chromatin (Papanicolaou, oil, ×100 objective)

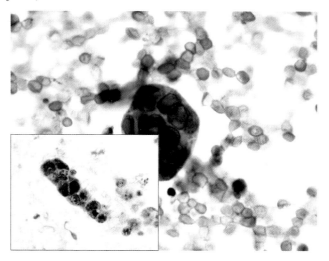

Fig. 4.2 *Herpes simplex*, in bronchial brush specimen (Papanicolaou, oil, × 100 objective). *Insert* shows Herpes simplex immunoreactivity in a cell block preparation. (Immunoperoxidase with diaminobenzidine (DAB) and hematoxylin, low power)

Differential diagnosis: Herpetic changes should be differentiated from CMV and other viruses, and from giant cells resulting
from chemotherapy or radiation therapy. CMV usually does not
appear in sheets but rather as isolated cells, and is less likely to
be associated with necrosis. Other viruses, including measles, display multinucleation similar to herpes, but these are rarely encountered in cytologic material, and immunocytochemical staining
will rule out herpes. Unlike those of herpes, cells associated
with chemotherapy or radiation show concomitant enlargement
of the cytoplasm and nucleus, and although multinucleation is
not uncommon, the nuclei are more centrally located rather than
occupying the entire cell, and they lack the characteristic molded
appearance. The chromatin is usually bland or coarsely clumped,
and it lacks a clearly defined central inclusion.

Cytomegalovirus Infection

Similar to herpes simplex, cytomegalovirus infection is more
common in immunocompromised patients. The virus affects
macrophages, pneumocytes, bronchial epithelial and endothelial
cells, but in view of the small numbers of the diagnostic cells,
the sensitivity of detection by BAL is only around 20–40%. The
scant characteristic cells encountered exhibit marked cytomegaly
associated with nucleomegaly. The cells usually possess one or
two nuclei that are centrally located and do not occupy the entire
cell, unlike those of herpes simplex. Two types of basophilic inclusions are encountered: intranuclear and cytoplasmic. The intranuclear inclusion is a single, large round basophilic structure with
a smooth contour, surrounded by a distinct clear halo, giving the
appearance of an "owl-eye." The nuclear rim is dense due to chromatin margination on its inner surface (Fig. 4.3). The cytoplasmic
inclusions are multiple, basophilic and vary in size, but are smaller
than the intranuclear ones. In addition to these characteristic CMV
cells, the cytologic preparation may include mixed inflammatory
cells and respiratory cells showing ciliocytophthoria or smudged
nuclei.

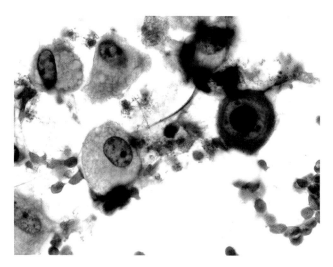

Fig. 4.3 Cytomegalovirus effects in sputum. There is enlargement of the nucleus and cytoplasm, with a large intranuclear inclusion surrounded by a halo. The cytoplasm contains smaller viral inclusions (Papanicolaou, oil, × 100 objective)

Key Features
- Marked cytomegaly and karyomegaly
- One or two large nuclei
- Cyanophilic intranuclear and cytoplasmic inclusions
- Nuclear inclusion is single, large with a halo (owl-eye)
- Cytoplasmic inclusions multiple, smaller and vary in size
- Ciliocytophthoria
- Mixed but often minimal inflammatory cells

Differential diagnosis: The nuclear size and location, cell size, as well as lack of sheets and necrosis help to differentiate *CMV* from *herpes simplex*. Neoplastic giant cells are usually seen in sheets or small clusters rather than as individual cells of *CMV*. Their nuclei exhibit marked nuclear pleomorphism and lack the characteristic inclusions of *CMV*. Immunocytochemistry is not usually needed to establish the diagnosis of *CMV*, but may be used for confirmation, particularly in cell block preparations, or when reactive epithelial cells or macrophages show karyomegaly. Other viruses, such as Respiratory Syncytial virus and Adenovirus should be excluded.

Adenovirus Infection

Infection of the bronchial epithelium with *adenovirus* results in cells with large smudgy nuclei, referred to as "smudge cells" which have small, multiple inclusions. In addition, a single small eosinophilic intranuclear inclusion may be seen, surrounded by a halo not unlike that of herpes. Adenovirus infection is often associated with ciliocytophthoria.

Other Viral Infections

Respiratory syncytial virus is often a cause of infection in children, and is not uncommonly identified in cytologic material in lung allograft recipients. Fusion of multiple cells results in syncytial giant cells with several nuclei and intracytoplasmic eosinophilic inclusions surrounded by clear halos. The cytoplasmic inclusions can also be seen in bronchial or alveolar cells. Influenza, though very common infection, is not associated with specific cytomorphologic viral changes. Parainfluenza and *Varicella zoster* have also been reported but have no pathognomonic cytomorphology.

Bacterial Infections

The role of cytopathology in the diagnosis of bacterial infections is usually limited, although some organisms, such as mycobacteria, often provide clues to their nature. Treatment depends on proper identification of organisms as well as determination of their sensitivity to antibiotics, parameters that require microbiologic culture and sensitivity tests. Examination of cytologic material, however, can be very helpful in differentiating infectious from neoplastic lesions, and ensuring adequate sampling for microbiologic studies. Appropriate triaging of samples in a timely fashion can also be facilitated when needle aspiration biopsy is combined with on-site evaluation.

Most bacterial pneumonias and abscesses are caused by a variety of Gram positive and Gram negative bacteria, and result in an abundance of neutrophils. The polymorphonuclear leucocytes are associated with cell debris, mixed with mucus and macrophages. This picture is altered if the patient is immunosuppressed; the inflammatory response may then be sparse or absent. A discussion of infections that produce some characteristic cytologic patterns follows.

Mycobacterial Infections

Tuberculosis continues to be a common disease, with several drug-resistant strains being recognized worldwide. The majority of cases are caused by *M. tuberculosis* and *M. avium intracellulare*. The cytologic manifestations are usually nonspecific, but the disease should be suspected in the presence of eosinophilic necrotic material, associated with histiocytic, neutrophilic and lymphocytic infiltrate. Multinucleated Langhans giant cells are encountered only in about 5% of sputum samples, but when identified they help to support the diagnosis. In needle aspirates, granulomas can be recognized by tight aggregates of histiocytes (epithelioid histiocytes), lymphocytes and fibroblasts around necrotic centers. Langhans giant cells are not always present. In some cases, one of these elements (necrosis, histiocytes or fibroblasts) is predominantly present (Figs. 4.4 and 4.5). Other organisms, however, can induce necrotizing granulomas with classic Langhans giant cells, as previously illustrated in the case of coccidioidomycosis (see Fig. 2.8). Attempts to identify the acid fast organisms by special stains such as Ziehl Neelsen (Fig. 4.6A) or auramine-rhodamine immunofluorescence may be successful, but microbiologic studies including culture and PCR, are more productive for cytologic material. Culture may require 12 weeks to produce definitive results, while PCR testing has the advantage of a short turn-around-time of only 2 days. If acid fast bacilli are identified by special stains but specific typing is not feasible, the term mycobacteriosis is used.

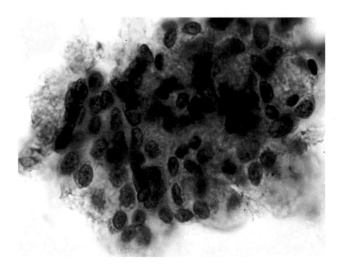

Fig. 4.4 Granulomatous reaction. There are aggregates of epithelioid histiocytes associated with necrosis in this sample from a patient with pulmonary
tuberculosis (Papanicolaou, high power)

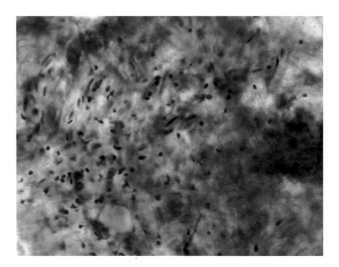

Fig. 4.5 Tuberculous granuloma. Note necrosis in background (Papanicolaou,
medium power)

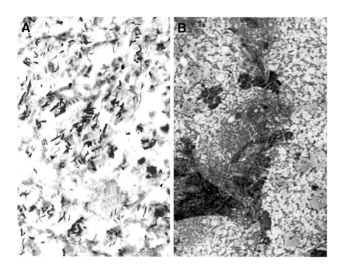

Fig. 4.6   Acid fast bacteria. (**A**) Acid fast stain showing many acid fast bacilli. The presence of large numbers of these bacilli is usually associated with immunocompromised settings (Ziehl Neelsen, oil, ×100 objective). (**B**) Mycobacterium avium intracellulare infection in an immunocompromised patient, demonstrating the negative staining of the organisms within the cytoplasm and in the background (Diff-Quik, oil, ×100 objective)

In immunocompromised patients the infection is overwhelming, with a large number of bacilli that fill the cytoplasm of macrophages. Since the bacilli do not stain with Papanicolaou or Diff-Quik stains, they appear as clear spaces due to the negative image they impart on the stained material (Fig. 4.6B). These cases, which are often caused by *M. avium*, frequently lack the inflammatory response, and Langhans giant cells are rarely encountered.

Key Features
- Eosinophilic necrotic material
- Lymphocytes and histiocytes
- Rare multinucleated Langhans cells (5%)
- Squamous cell atypia in chronic cases
- Abundant bacilli with negative images in immunodeficiency
- Inflammatory response lacking if immunocompromised

Differential diagnosis: Chronic tuberculous infection may induce squamous metaplasia, and marked nuclear atypia that can mimic carcinoma (see Fig. 7.12). Careful attention to nuclear features and clinical data help to avoid overcalling such cells. Tuberculosis should also be differentiated from other granulomatous lesions, such as fungal infections, rheumatoid granuloma and Wegener granulomatosis. Nocardia can also produce negative images on Diff-Quik preparations, but the filamentous organisms are extracellular. Sarcoidosis produces noncaseating granulomas and should be considered in the differential diagnosis; the lack of necrotic debris, however, supports the diagnosis of sarcoid in the proper clinical setting.

Legionella Infection

Two organisms, *L. pneumophila* and *L. micdadei* can be responsible for some cases of pneumonia. The resulting neutrophilic inflammatory exudate has no specific cytologic characteristics, but the organisms appear as small Gram negative rods that stain with Dieterle silver or fluorescent antibody stains, and the disease can be easily diagnosed by serologic testing.

Actinomycosis and Nocardiosis

Actinomyces colonies are frequently seen in tonsillar crypts and other parts of the oral cavity, particularly in persons with poor oral hygiene. Their presence in sputum indicates contamination from oral contents. However, they are significant if encountered in BAL or FNA specimens from a lung mass, particularly in immunocompromised individuals (Fig. 4.7). The organisms form colonies of thin beaded and delicate branching filaments that are cyanophilic with Papanicolaou stain. They occasionally display eosinophilic club ends at the periphery of the colony, a manifestation of the Splendore-Hoeppli phenomenon. Actinomyces are acid fast organisms and they stain positively with GMS. Nocardia shares the same morphology as Actinomyces, but is only weakly acid fast with modified stains such as Fite's. Both organisms can

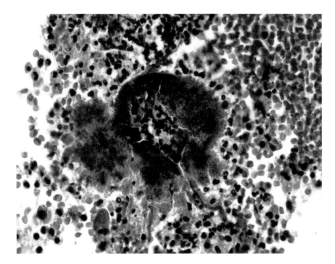

Fig. 4.7 Actinomycosis colony. Cell block preparation from a fine needle aspirate of a mass that proved to be an abscess. Note the peripheral clubbing and the neutrophilic exudate (H & E, medium power)

also induce reactive hyperplasia in terminal bronchioles and pneumocytes (see Fig. 3.5).

Other Bacteria

Many species of bacteria, other than those described above, can be associated with upper and lower respiratory tract infections, and often one infection is superimposed on another caused by a second organism. This is particularly true in the case of immunosuppressed or elderly patients. *Rhodococcus equi*, an example of such rare infections, is a small pleomorphic Gram positive coccobacillus that has a tendency to be associated with malakoplakia.

Mycotic Infections

Mycotic infections often involve the respiratory organs, particularly in immunosuppressed individuals, such as in AIDS and transplant patients. Cytologic examination can be quite helpful in the early detection of these infections. Although fungal infections can result in nonspecific granulomatous response, similar to that of mycobacteriosis, some cytomorphologic features can help identify the causative fungus. The diagnosis can be further supported with the use of special fungal stains such as GMS or PAS, in addition to the more elaborate microbiologic testing such as culture and PCR.

Candidiasis

Candida organisms are normally encountered in the oral cavity and may colonize the upper respiratory tract, and similar to Actinomyces, are asymptomatic in immunocompetent patients. These organisms, however, are a common cause of opportunistic infections in immunocompromised patients. True infections are usually associated with an acute inflammatory response of neutrophils. The fungal organisms of *Candida albicans* appear as pseudohyphae or budding yeast (blastoconidia) forms. The pseudoseptate hyphae have an irregular diameter of approximately 10–15 μm (Fig. 4.8A, B). These are associated with isolated clusters of 2- to 4-μm oval or teardrop yeast forms, some of which may be budding from the pseudohyphae. The pseudohyphae and spores stain yellowish brown with the Papanicolaou stain. Nuclear atypia of the squamous cells may be encountered, but it is usually slight. The inflammatory background and the close association of the atypical cells with characteristic organisms help in establishing the benign nature of atypia.

Key Features
- Opportunistic infection
- Pseudohyphae irregular in diameter (10–15 μm)
- Yeast buds oval or teardrop, 2–4 μm
- Nuclear atypia of squamous cells near organisms

Differential diagnosis: Candida organisms are often encountered in specimens that are contaminated with oral contents by various mechanisms, including the introduction of the

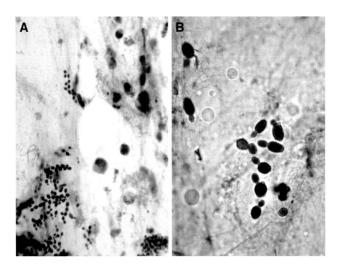

Fig. 4.8 *Candida albicans.* (**A**) The organisms appear in sputum as clusters of yeast forms; oral contamination should be considered in less than optimal specimens (medium power). (**B**) Higher magnification reveals the budding yeast (Papanicolaou, Oil, ×100 objective)

bronchoscope through the oral cavity. It may be difficult to determine the significance of their presence in the procured material in the absence of any clinical data indicating respiratory infection. The association of large numbers of benign superficial squamous cells favors the oral cavity as the source of the organisms. Other causes of pneumonia should be excluded prior to attributing the manifestations to Candidiasis. Candida should be differentiated from other fungi, particularly Aspergillus, Histoplasma, Cryptococcus and Blastomyces by the characteristic morphology, size, pattern of branching and intra or extracellular location of the organisms.

Cryptococcosis

Cryptococcus infections are uncommon, except in debilitated or immunocompromised individuals. The infection can be systemic and overwhelming in such setting, with involvement of lymph nodes, visceral organs particularly lungs, as well as meninges. The accompanying inflammatory response is often mild or lacking, although large number of organisms can be encountered. These infections are caused by *Cryptococcus neoformans*, an organism found in soil contaminated with bird droppings, and seen worldwide, particularly in Western United States and Australia. The budding yeast is an encapsulated mostly round to slightly oval organism, with marked variation in diameter (5–20 μm). The fungal organisms are GMS positive, and are surrounded by a characteristically thick mucoid capsule. With Papanicolaou stain, the capsule appears as a well defined pale or clear space around the central slightly refractile pale brown organism. Mucicarmine and PAS, however, stain the thick capsule, thus the apparent larger diameter of the fungus with these stains (Figs. 4.9A, B and 4.10 A, B). A single spore may be seen attached to the parent organism by a narrow "tear-drop" base.

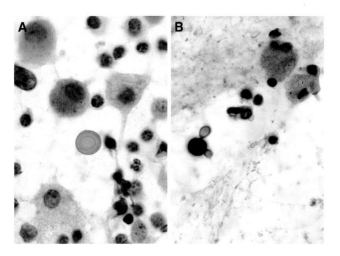

Fig. 4.9 *Cryptococcus neoformans* in sputum in a patient undergoing treatment. (**A**) The organisms show variation in size under such circumstances (Papanicolaou, Oil, ×100 objective). (**B**) Tear drop buds are evident in this preparation (Diff-Quik, oil, ×100 objective)

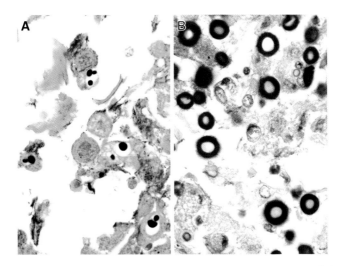

Fig. 4.10 *Cryptococcus neoformans*. (**A**) Organisms stain with Gomori silver methenamine, surrounded by a halo representing the thick mucoid capsule (GMS, oil, ×100 objective). (**B**) The organisms appear larger with mucicarmine which stains the thick mucoid capsule (Mucicarmine, oil, ×100 objective)

Key Features
- Often in immunocompromised patients
- Round to slightly oval yeast
- Marked size variation (5–20 μm)
- Thick mucoid mucicarmine and PAS positive capsule
- Single tear drop like spore

Differential diagnosis: Blastomycetes are less commonly encountered than cryptococci. They lack the thick mucoid capsule of Cryptococcus, and have a single bud that is broad based. *Histoplasma capsulatum* shares some morphologic features with *C. neoformans*, particularly when the latter is a capsule-deficient variant. Histoplasma organisms, however, tend to be smaller and are located within the cytoplasm of histiocytes, while *C. neoformans* is only rarely seen within Langhans giant cells in cytologic specimens.

Aspergillosis

Inhalation of the spores of Aspergillus spp. produces a variety of pulmonary lesions, especially in immunosuppressed individuals. The spectrum of lesions includes localized mycetoma (aspergilloma), diffuse invasive aspergillosis, abscesses, eosinophilic pneumonia or allergic bronchopulmonary aspergillosis (ABPA). The spores of *A. fumigatus*, *A. flavus*, or *A. niger* are 4 μm in diameter. In tissues, the organism forms septate hyphae that are 3–6 μm in diameter and branch dichotomously at an acute 45° angle. These can be identified in BAL, sputum or FNA cytologic material, particularly with the help of GMS staining (Fig. 4.11A, B). Aspergillus may form a granuloma that contains a fungus ball within air-containing cavities or in large airways. This is referred to as an aspergilloma, and fruiting heads (conidiophores) may be developing in such environment (Fig. 4.12A, B). Birefringent calcium oxalate crystals may

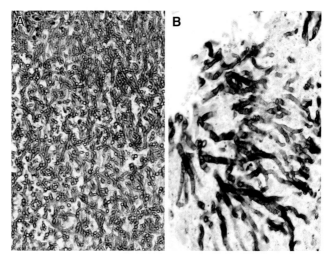

Fig. 4.11 Aspergillosis. (**A**) Cell block preparation from an FNA of a lung mass showing a colony of *A. niger* resulting in an aspergilloma. (H & E, medium power). (**B**) The organisms of the aspergilloma show uniform thickness and branching at acute angles. Compare to Fig. 4.15 of zygomycetes (GMS, high power)

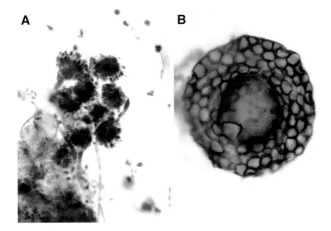

Fig. 4.12 Aspergillosis. (**A**) Conidiophores (fruiting bodies) only appear in cavities that contain air. Such cavities produce a characteristic air level on imaging (Papanicolaou, medium power), Slide courtesy of Azam Alizadeh, CT, Houston, TX. (**B**) Aspergillus fruiting head from a paranasal sinus (Papanicolaou, high power)

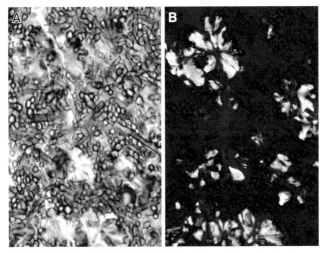

Fig. 4.13 Oxalate crystals associated with *A. niger*. (**A**) Crystals appear in this BAL material as faint structures when examined under ordinary microscopic light (H & E, high power). (**B**) Same preparation as in (A) seen under polarized light clearly demonstrates the refractile crystals. (H & E, high power, polarized light)

be identified under polarized light in *A. niger* infections, but these crystals were also observed in other mycotic infections (Fig. 4.13A, B). The morphologic characteristics of the fungus can be altered in treated cases, with marked variation in the diameter of hyphae and weak staining of the necrotic organisms. Allergic bronchopulmonary aspergillosis produces a characteristic clinical pattern, with peripheral eosinophilia. The cytologic material in such cases may demonstrate eosinophils and Charcot–Leyden crystals. One of the features suggestive of aspergillosis is the tendency of mucous plugs to appear as "onion-skin like" layers of mucus mixed with inflammatory cells (Fig. 4.14).

Key Features
- Septate hyphae with dichotomous branching at 45°
- Diameter 3–6 μm, uniform unless treated
- Calcium oxalate crystals
- Granulomatous reaction
- Eosinophils and lamellated mucus in ABPA
- Treatment induces variation in diameter

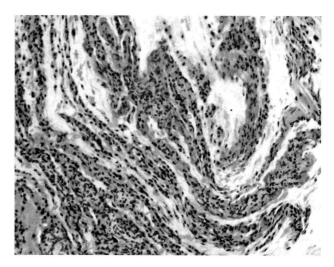

Fig. 4.14 Mucus plug in Allergic Bronchopulmonary Aspergillosis (ABPA). The plugs often have characteristic laminations of mucus (H & E, low power)

Differential diagnosis: Zygomycosis is characterized by broad hyphae that branch at right angles. *Candida albicans* show pseudo-hyphae and yeast forms. Fusarium exhibits cytomorphology that overlaps with Aspergillus, and it has been reported as a cause of disseminated infection in immunocompromised patients. Culture and sensitivity testing is essential in establishing the proper classification of such organisms.

Zygomycosis (Phycomycosis)

These ubiquitous fungi, commonly present as molds, are sometimes encountered in paranasal sinuses and are usually asymptomatic in immunocompetent persons. When the patient's immunity is compromised, however, these fungi can be a serious threat to life, since they have a tendency to rapid vascular invasion, causing thrombosis and its serious sequelae. The broad ribbon-like nonseptate hyphae exhibit marked variation in diameter (6–50 μm.) and they branch at right angles (Fig. 4.15).

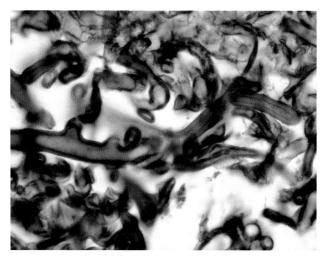

Fig. 4.15   Zygomycosis. The ribbon-like organisms have thick walls and branch at 90° angles (Papanicolaou, oil, ×100 objective)

Occasionally the nonseptate hyphae fold and wrinkle, giving a false impression of septation. In contrast, Aspergillus hyphae are thin, truly septate and they branch at 45°. Both organisms may coexist, particularly as commensals in the upper respiratory tract.

Key Features
- Broad nonseptate hyphae
- Branching at 90°
- Marked variation in diameter (6–50 μm)
- Immunocompromised patients

Histoplasmosis

This is encountered in many parts of the world, usually as a result of inhaling soil infested with bird droppings. *H. capsulatum* is the organism seen in the Americas, including the Ohio and Mississippi valleys, while the slightly larger *H. duboisii* is the African variant. The organism induces a necrotizing granulomatous reaction with formation of coin lesions, but in immunosuppressed patients, the infection can be overwhelming, not unlike tuberculosis. The organism is a small uninucleate fungus, 2–4 μm diameter that is mostly encountered within macrophages, neutrophils and also extracellularly in areas of necrosis (Fig. 4.16). The capsule stains with GMS and PAS, while the center stains with Giemsa or Diff-Quik.

Key Features
- Often asymptomatic, unless in immunocompromised patient
- Organisms mostly intracellular, 2–4 μm in diameter each
- Thin PAS and GMS positive capsule
- Seen within macrophages and neutrophils
- Granulomatous reaction with extracellular organisms

Differential diagnosis: *Leishmania spp*. has kinetoplasts that are evident by Giemsa stain, their capsule is PAS negative and there is no granulomatous response. *C. neoformans* organisms are

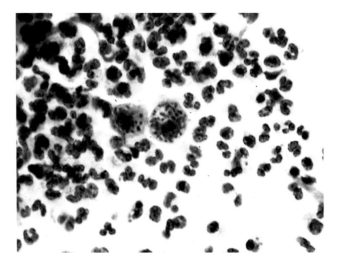

Fig. 4.16 Histoplasmosis. The small organisms are seen within the cytoplasm of macrophages. Note the inflammatory response in the background (Papanicolaou, high power)

mostly extracellular, have a thick mucoid capsule and are larger than *H. capsulatum.*

Blastomycosis

Blastomyces dermatiditis infection is more common in the Southeast United States as well as the Ohio and Mississippi River valleys. It involves the skin, lungs and other organs where it evokes a granulomatous response. Examination of sputum, lavage or needle biopsy specimens may demonstrate the fungus within histiocytes or in necrotic background material. *B. dermatiditis* appears as uniform round 8–20 μm yeast, with thick refractile double contoured wall. A characteristic broad-based bud that is 4–5 μm in diameter differentiates this fungus from cryptococcus organisms (Fig. 4.17).

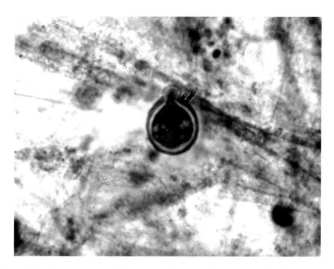

Fig. 4.17 Blastomycosis. The patient had a skin lesion on his leg and pulmonary consolidation. Sputum material demonstrated the round to slightly oval organisms, with a single bud that had a broad-based bud. Compare to the bud in cryptococcus organisms in Fig. 4.9B (Papanicolaou, oil, ×100 objective). Case courtesy Dr. Ian Turnbull, London, Ontario, Canada

Key Features
- Uniform round 8–20 μm, within macrophages or in necrotic debris
- Thick refractile wall
- Broad-based bud 4–5 μm

Coccidiodomycosis and Paracoccidiodomycosis

Coccidioides immitis is endemic to the southwestern United States, northern Mexico and parts of Central and South America. Although some patients develop clinically significant pulmonary disease, two thirds of individuals are asymptomatic or show only transient respiratory symptoms. The causative organisms appear as large (20–100 μm diameter) sporangia (endosporulating spherules) that contain variable numbers of endospores, each of which is 1–5 μm in diameter. The sporangia may be

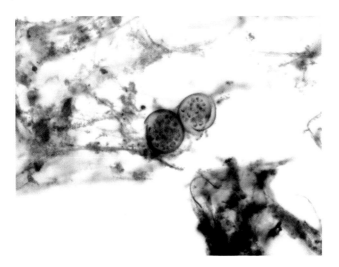

Fig. 4.18 Coccidioidomycosis. A transbronchial FNA material procured from a lung mass. The cyst contains a large number of sporangia which stain red. (Papanicolaou, high power)

free in necrotic material or within multinucleated giant histiocytes (Figs. 4.18 and 4.19). They stain positively with GMS and PAS. Hyphae rarely form and usually only in cavitary lesions.

Key Features
- Organisms in giant cells or necrotic background
- Large sporangia (20–100 μm) containing endospores
- Endospores are 1–5 μm in diameter
- Hyphae exceptionally rare

Paracoccidioides brasiliensis, also known as *Blastomyces brasiliensis*, is endemic to South America. It is characterized by multiple buds that surround the central fungus, giving it a "pilot's wheel" appearance that is 5–40 μm in diameter. The organisms induce granulomatous and giant cell reaction. When the fungal bodies lack the characteristic buds, differentiation from *Coccidioides immitis* and Blastomyces can be difficult, since they also share the same staining characteristics.

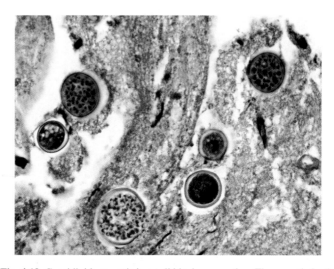

Fig. 4.19 Coccidioidomycosis in a cell block preparation. The necrotic background material surrounds several sporangia, some containing endospores (H & E, high power). See also Fig. 2.8

Sporotrichosis

Sporotrichosis is worldwide in distribution, usually involving skin and subcutaneous tissues. However, it can cause systemic disease involving the lungs and other internal organs, particularly in mildly immunosuppressed patients such as diabetics. The lesions are pyogranulomatous, with organisms seen free or within giant cells. *Sporotrichum (Sporothrix) schenckii* appears as small (3–6 μm) yeast forms, with one or more tear-drop buds. Morphologic differentiation from other small fungi such as Histoplasma, Cryptococcus, or Candida can be difficult, and cultures may be necessary.

Pneumocystis jiroveci (carinii) Pneumonia

Pneumocystis jiroveci is becoming a major cause of pneumonia in immunosuppressed patients, particularly those with AIDS. Bronchoalveolar lavage is frequently used to detect this infection;

its sensitivity is around 90–98%. There has been a longstanding debate regarding the nature of *Pneumocystis jiroveci*, but ribosomal RNA sequences support classifying it as a fungus rather than protozoa. In respiratory material, particularly BAL specimens stained with the Papanicolaou technique, the alveolar contents appear as cyanophilic or purple frothy material which consists of secretions mixed with the organisms (Fig. 4.20). The latter appear as tiny basophilic dots within the spaces of the foamy exudate. With silver stains, such as GMS, the organisms appear as small (6–8 μm) spherical, wrinkled, crescent or cup-shaped capsules that look like crushed ping-pong balls (Fig. 4.21). In Papanicolaou stained material, *P. jiroveci* cysts show fluorescence when viewed under ultraviolet light. Within these cysts, one or more tiny basophilic structures may be evident. These structures, originally considered trophozoites, can also be visualized by metachromatic stains such as Diff-Quik, Giemsa or Toluidine blue. Although the frothy exudate is fairly characteristic, it may be absent and in such

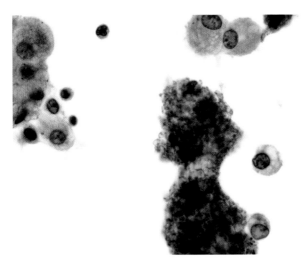

Fig. 4.20 *Pneumocystis jiroveci* in AIDS. In smears stained with Papanicolaou stain, the organisms appear as small dots within a characteristic fluffy cotton like background material (Papanicolaou, high power)

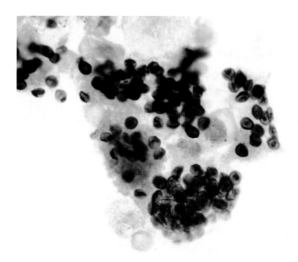

Fig. 4.21 *Pneumocystis jiroveci.* The organisms are easy to detect in GMS stained preparations, appearing as fragile punched "ping pong balls" and a few structures may be identified in the center of the cysts (GMS, oil, ×100 objective)

cases, direct fluorescent antibody stains for the organism may be helpful. In many cases, there is minimal inflammatory reaction, diffuse alveolar damage or a granulomatous reaction to *P. jiroveci* infection.

Key Features
- Frothy background containing organisms
- Crescent or cup shaped 6–8 μm, cysts
- One or more minute basophilic "dots" within the cysts
- GMS stains cyst wall, Diff-Quik or Giemsa stain the dots
- Patient is usually immunocompromised
- Inflammatory reaction minimal, if any

Differential diagnosis: Mucin aggregates lack the tiny dots that represent *P. jiroveci* organisms on Papanicolaou-stained slides. With GMS, mucin stains diffusely and lacks the characteristic cysts of *P. jiroveci.* Pulmonary alveolar proteinosis results in dense glob-ules of eosinophilic exudate that appears to be hard rather than frothy, and lacks the characteristic organisms by GMS. Cases of alveolar proteinosis, however, have been reported in patients recovering from *P. jiroveci* pneumonia. When *P. jiroveci* organisms are sparse, they can be differentiated from poorly stained red blood cells and yeast by the characteristic structures within the cysts.

Parasitic Infections

Several parasites may reach the lung, and result in allergic response. Some of these produce specific patterns that help in identifying the causative parasite. These include Strongyloides, Schistosoma, Paragonimus, amoeba among others.

Strongyloidiasis

Strongyloidiasis has worldwide distribution, and is endemic in southern United States. Strongyloides stercoralis life cycle includes a transient, often asymptomatic pulmonary phase. However, an overwhelming superinfestation of the lung is encountered in individuals who are immunosuppressed such as in AIDS, hematologic malignancies, prolonged steroid therapy and in transplant patients. In such cases, the rhabditiform larvae metamorphose into filariform larvae, penetrate the intestinal wall, migrate into blood vessels and ultimately reach the lungs. They induce pneumonic consolidation (Löffler syndrome) with eosinophilic reaction and hemorrhage. Sputum, tracheal aspirates and BAL material procured from these patients may demonstrate a large number of filariform, often curved larvae that are 400–500 μm long (Figs. 4.22 and 4.23). The characteristic notched tail is unlike the tapering tail of hookworm larvae.

Key Features
- Curved filariform larvae 400–500 μm long
- Notched tail
- Superinfestation if immunocompromised
- Eosinophilic reaction in background

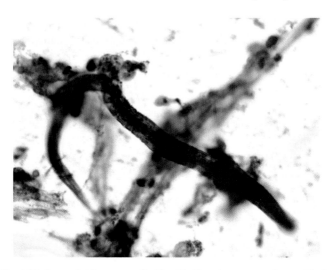

Fig. 4.22 *Strongyloides stercoralis*. The filariform larvae were detected in the sputum of a patient undergoing chemotherapy. The nematode has a characteristic tail notch (Papanicolaou, medium power)

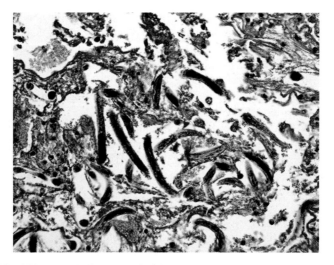

Fig. 4.23 *Strongyloides stercoralis*. The large number of filariform larvae seen in the cell block reflects a superinfestation in a patient suffering from AIDS (H & E, low power)

Differential diagnosis: *Ascaris lumbricoides* and hookworms also involve the lungs in their larval stage of their life cycle, but are unlikely to cause severe manifestations of pulmonary superinfestation and do not appear in BALs or sputa. Their larvae lack the characteristic tail notch.

Paragonimiasis

This disease is much more prevalent in the Far East than in the United States, and is most frequently caused by *Paragonimus westermani* (lung fluke). The metacercaria, excyst in the intestine, migrate through the liver and peritoneum and eventually reach the lung where they mature. They induce allergic and granulomatous response, abscesses, cysts and calcification. If the golden brown operculated eggs reach an airway, they can appear in the sputum or bronchial washings. They can also be seen in FNA specimens, often associated with a prominent eosinophilic infiltrate and Charcot–Leyden crystals. (Fig. 4.24A and B).

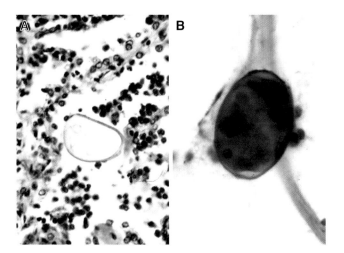

Fig. 4.24 Paragonimiasis. (**A**) A fine needle aspirate of a pulmonary lesion showing an inflammatory response surrounding the ovum (medium power). (**B**) The ovum is operculated (Papanicolaou, high power). Case courtesy of Dr. Uei, Tokyo, Japan

Dirofilariasis

Pulmonary dirofilarisis is caused by *Dirofilaria immitis* (dog heartworm) and has been reported mostly in the southern United States. The worm dies in the human heart and can then cause pulmonary thrombus and infarct. Although mostly asymptomatic, it can cause a radiologically-alarming coin lesion that mimics carcinoma. FNA material demonstrates the necrotic worm surrounded by a granulomatous reaction with eosinophils, plasma cells, histiocytes and giant cells.

Other Parasitic Infections

Cases of pulmonary involvement by Echinococcus, Amoeba, Schistosoma, Toxoplasma, Cryptosporidium, Microfilaria, and Trichomonas organisms have been reported. A detailed description of these is beyond the scope of this text.

Suggested Reading

Viral

Bayon MN, Drut R. Cytologic diagnosis of adenovirus bronchopneumonia. Acta Cytol 1991;35:181–182

Bower M, Baron SW, Nelson MR, et al. The significance of detection of cytomegalovirus in the bronchoalveolar lavage fluids in AIDS patients with pneumonia. AIDS 1990;4:317–332

Crosby JH, Pantazis CG, Stigall B. In situ DNA hybridization for confirmation of Herpes simplex virus in bronchoalveolar lavage smears. Acta Cytol 1991;35:248–250

Harboldt SL, Dugan JM, Tronic BS. Cytologic diagnosis of measles pneumonia in a bronchoalveolar lavage specimen. A case report. Acta Cytol 1994;38:403–406

Lapkus O, Elsheikh TM, Ujevich BA, et al. Pitfalls in the diagnosis of herpes simplex infection in respiratory cytology. Acta Cytol 2006;50:617–620

Lemert CM, Baughman RP, Hayner CE, et al. Relationship between cytomegalovirus cells and survival in acquired immunodeficiency syndrome patients. Acta Cytol 1996;40:205–210

Parham DM, Bozeman P, Killian C, et al. Cytologic diagnosis of respiratory syncytial virus infection in a bronchoalveolar lavage specimen from a bone marrow transplant recipient. Am J Clin Pathol 1993;99:588–592

Pierce CH, Knox AW. Ciliocytophthoria in sputum from patients with adenovirus infections. Proc Soc Exp Biol Med 1960;104:492–495

Zaman SS, Seykora JT, Hodinka RL, et al. Cytologic manifestations of respiratory syncytial virus pneumonia in bronchoalveolar lavage fluid. Acta Cytol 1996;l40:546–551

Bacterial

Das DK, Bhambhani S, Pant JN, et al. Superficial and deep-seated tuberculous lesions: fine needle aspiration cytology diagnosis of 574 cases. Diag Cytopathol 1989;8:211–215

Hsu C-Y, Luh K-T. Cytology of pulmonary Fusobacterium nucleatum infection. Acta Cytol 1995;39:114–117

Lachman MF. Cytologic appearance of Rhodococcus equi in bronchoalveolar lavage specimens. Acta Cytol 1995;39:111–113

Trisolini R, Paioli D, Patelli M, et al. Brochoalveolar lavage. Intact granulomas in Mycobacterium avium pulmonary infection. Acta Cytol 2008;52:263–264

Fungal

Chen KTK. Cytology of allergic bronchopulmonary aspergillosis. Diagn Cytopathol 1993;9:82–85

Chen KT. Cytodiagnostic pitfalls in pulmonary coccidioidomycosis. Diagn Cytopathol 1995;12:177–180

Fraire AE, Kemp B, Greenberg SD, et al. Calclflor white stain for the detection of Pneumocystis carinii in transbronchial lung biopsy specimens: a study of 68 cases. Mod Pathol 1996;9:861–864

Hsu CY. Cytologic diagnosis of pulmonary cryptococcosis in immunocompetent hosts. Acta Cytol 1993;37:667–672

Johnston WW, Amatulli J. The role of cytology in the primary diagnosis of North American blastomycosis. Acta Cytol 1970;14:200–204

Raab SS, Silverman JF, Zimmerman KG. Fine-needle aspiration biopsy of pulmonary coccidioidomycosis. Spectrum of cytologic findings in 73 patients. Am J Clin Pathol 1993;99:582–587

Parasitic

Rangdaeng S, Alpert LC, Khiyama A. Pulmonary paragonimiasis. Report
of a case with diagnosis by fine needle aspiration cytology. Acta Cytol
1992;36:31–36

Ro JY, Tsakalakis PJ, White VA, et al. Pulmonary dirofilariasis. The great
imitator of primary or metastatic lung tumor. A clinico-pathologic analysis
of seven cases and review of the literature. Hum Pathol 1989;20:69–76

Chapter 5
Other Nonneoplastic Conditions

Bronchial Asthma

Allergens induce a reaction characterized by hyperplasia of the columnar ciliated and mucinous cells lining the bronchial tree and plugging of small bronchi by inspissated mucin. Cytologic material shows sheets or tightly cohesive three-dimensional fragments of hypersecretory respiratory epithelium with goblet cells and ciliated columnar cells, referred to as "Creola bodies." Abundant mucus is present in the background, and casts of small bronchi and bronchioles, in the form of Curschmann spirals, are often identified. Increased numbers of eosinophils is a reflection of the allergic nature of the disease. This is associated with the presence of Charcot–Leyden crystals which result from crystallization of the protein in the cytoplasm of eosinophils (Fig. 5.1).

Key Features
- Clusters of hyperplastic ciliated columnar epithelial cells
- Hyperplastic goblet cells
- Abundant mucus in background
- Curschmann spirals
- Eosinophils and Charcot–Leyden crystals

Differential diagnosis: The difficulty in visualizing nuclear features in the three dimensional clusters of hyperplastic epithelium may lead to erroneous interpretation as being derived from an

Y.S. Erozan, I. Ramzy, *Pulmonary Cytopathology*,
Essentials in Cytopathology 6, DOI 10.1007/978-0-387-88888-0_5,
© Springer Science+Business Media, LLC 2009

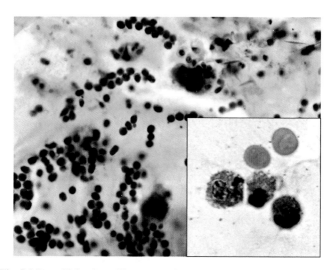

Fig. 5.1 Bronchial asthma. The sputum shows an eosinophilic infiltrate, mucus and Charcot–Leyden crystals. *Inset* shows the granules in eosinophils which may stain brown in Papanicolaou stained smears (Papanicolaou, medium power, *inset* at high power). See also Fig. 2.11A, B and Fig. 2.12

adenocarcinoma. However, examination of these bodies at different levels of focus, particularly with a partially closed microscope condenser, reveals preservation of some cilia or terminal bars at the edge of the cluster or in its central core. Another source of difficulty is the presence of precipitated mucus that may simulate crushed cells of small cell carcinoma. Search for intact cells with clear malignant features in their nuclei, rather than the structureless mucin deposit, clarifies the issue.

Sarcoidosis

Sarcoidosis is a systemic granulomatous disease, possibly resulting from altered immune reaction to an unknown agent, in a genetically predisposed background. It involves the lungs and mediastinal lymph nodes in 90% of cases. The cytologic findings are those of lymphocytic alveolitis and a granulomatous reaction. There is an increase in the number of lymphocytes, mostly

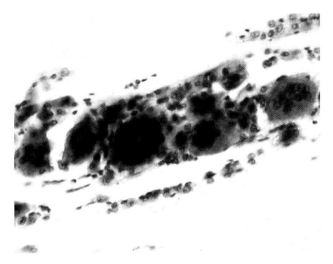

Fig. 5.2 Sarcoidosis. A bronchial brush material shows histiocytic aggregates and giant cells with focal calcification (Papanicolaou, medium power)

T-helper cells, with T-Helper to T-Suppressor ratio in BAL specimens increasing from 2:1 to 6:1. The histiocytic granulomas are similar to tuberculosis, but they are noncaseating and the epithelioid cells are not associated with necrotic debris (Figs. 5.2 and 5.3). Giant cells containing the star-shaped crystalloid "asteroid bodies" or concentric calcific "Schaumann bodies" are rarely encountered in cytologic material (Figs. 5.4 and 5.5). Their presence is suggestive but not diagnostic of the disease, since they can be encountered in other conditions. The diagnosis of sarcoidosis rests on clinical, radiologic and serologic findings, and FNA aspirates should be reported as "consistent with sarcoid-type granuloma," after exclusion of other causes of noncaseating granulomatous lesions, such as fungal infections, by special stains.

Key Features
- Granulomatous response
- Absence of necrosis
- Giant cells with asteroid bodies rare
- Schaumann calcified bodies rare
- Diagnosis by exclusion using special stains

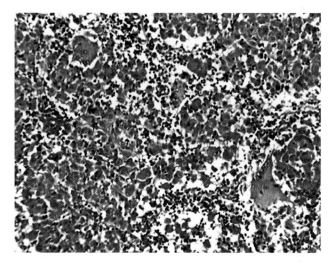

Fig. 5.3 Sarcoidosis. A cell block preparation from a transtracheal FNA shows epithelioid histiocytes, lymphocytes and some giant cells (H & E, low power)

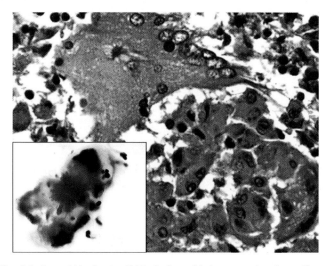

Fig. 5.4 Asteroid body. A cell block shows histiocytes and a giant cell containing asteroid body (H & E, high power). *Inset* shows an asteroid body with Papanicolaou stain

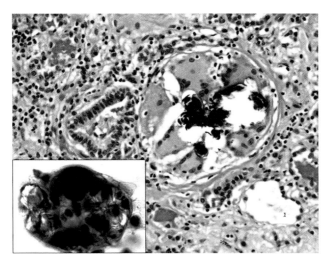

Fig. 5.5 Sarcoidosis with calcification. Cell block from an FNA of a hilar lesion (H & E, low power). *Inset* shows a calcified Schaumann bodies in a giant cell (Papanicolaou, medium power)

Pulmonary Alveolar Proteinosis

This condition is most commonly idiopathic. However, it can occur as a result of inhaling very fine dust, especially silica, altered immune reaction or in patients with hematologic malignancies. The alveolar spaces are full of a granular, dense globular proteinaceous material that contains deactivated lysosomal surfactant. Bronchoalveolar lavage is used for diagnosis and therapy. It results in procurement of a turbid fluid containing hyaline globular deposits. These deposits and granular background that are orangeophilic or cyanophilic are strongly positive with periodic acid-Schiff stain and are diastase resistant. Granular, PAS positive material is also seen in the cytoplasm of histiocytes and in the background (Figs. 5.6 and 5.7 A, B). Since the globules represent casts of the alveolar spaces, an occasional pneumocyte may be seen at their edge, hugging the globule.

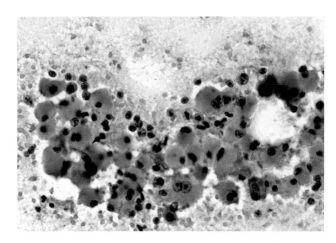

Fig. 5.6 Pulmonary alveolar proteinosis. Abundant pulmonary macrophages are seen in a background of eosinophilic granular material (H & E, medium power)

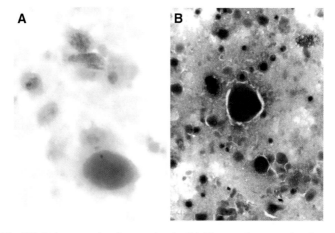

Fig. 5.7 Pulmonary alveolar proteinosis. (**A**) The proteinaceous deactivated surfactant within the alveoli forms cyanophilic globules (Papanicolaou, high power). (**B**) Positive staining of the globules with periodic acid Schiff is diastase resistant. (PAS with diastase digestion, medium power)

Key Features
- Bilateral involvement
- Hyaline globular eosinophilic or basophilic material
- Strong positive staining with PAS, diastase-resistant
- Type II pneumocytes at surface of globule

Differential diagnosis: The exudate in *Pneumocystis jiroveci* infection is foamy and loosely structured. It contains tiny dot-like structures representing the organisms. The clinical setting and GMS stains help to confirm the diagnosis.

Lipid Pneumonia

This reactive process is in response to exogenous or endogenous lipid material. Exogenous factors include inhalation of lipids such as mineral oil and nasal drops. Exogenous lipid pneumonia is characterized by a large number of macrophages with large well defined cytoplasmic vacuoles that vary in size. The vacuoles are strongly positive with oil red O, and are mucin-negative (Fig. 5.8). Occasionally, slight nuclear atypia is observed, and an acute or chronic inflammatory response may accompany the histiocytic reaction. Endogenous lipid pneumonia occurs in association with inflammatory lesions such as bronchitis obliterans organizing pneumonia (BOOP), idiopathic pulmonary fibrosis, bronchiectasis as well as in proximity of necrotic tissue or distal to an obstructive malignancy. In such cases, macrophages tend to have a fine stippled foamy cytoplasm.

Key Features
- Abundant macrophages
- Large sharply defined vacuoles if exogenous
- Cytoplasmic vacuoles more foamy if endogenous
- Vacuoles are Oil red O positive, mucin negative
- Nuclear atypia is slight

Differential diagnosis: In adenocarcinoma, the vacuoles are mucin positive, nuclear atypia is prominent and some epithelial

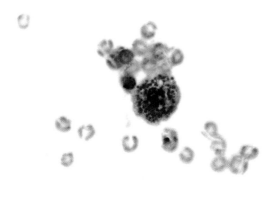

Fig. 5.8 Lipid pneumonia. The lipid material within a pulmonary macrophage is Oil Red O positive (Oil Red O, oil ×100 objective)

sheets or fragments can be identified. However, the two lesions can coexist, since it is not uncommon to see lipid pneumonia in association with necrotic areas of malignant tumors.

Amyloidosis

Amyloid deposits may involve the bronchial mucosa or the pulmonary parenchyma in a diffuse or nodular pattern. The sharply defined waxy, amorphous, acellular material may be encountered in BAL specimens or aspirates from large nodular lesions, but rarely in bronchial brush specimens or sputa. On Papanicolaou stained smears, they have a blue-green color (Fig. 5.9). They stain positively with Congo red and have a characteristic apple-green birefringence under polarized light (Figs. 5.10 and 5.11). Nodular amyloid deposits may also induce a foreign body giant cell reaction that often includes plasma cells.

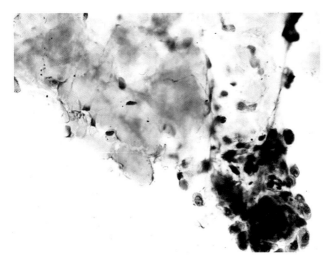

Fig. 5.9 Amyloidosis. The background shows cyanophilic homogeneous material (Papanicolaou, medium power)

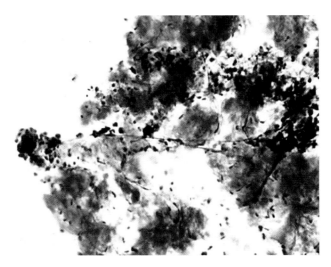

Fig. 5.10 Amyloidosis: Congo red stain depicts the amyloid material (Papanicolaou, low power)

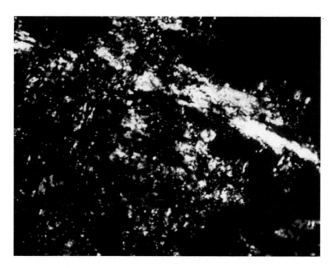

Fig. 5.11 Amyloidosis. Amyloid deposits show a characteristic apple green birefringence when the Congo red preparation is viewed under polarized light (Congo red, polarized light, low power)

Pulmonary Infarcts

Cytologic sampling of pulmonary infarcts occurs in two settings. The first is when a peripheral solitary consolidation mimics a neoplasm and FNA is necessary to rule out malignancy. The other clinical setting is when cytologic material is procured by bronchial brush or lavage from a patient with respiratory symptoms. Regardless of the pathogenetic mechanism, ischemia induces reactive changes in bronchial, alveolar and metaplastic squamous cells, with marked nuclear atypia that can be misinterpreted as evidence of malignancy. The ischemic atypia is characterized by tight clustering of the atypical cells, with enlarged hyperchromatic nuclei, irregular clearing and homogenization of nuclear chromatin and large prominent nucleoli. There is poor preservation or complete loss of cell walls leading to syncytiallike arrangement, with loss of nuclear detail. Additionally, the background often has blood and an abundance of hemosiderin-laden macrophages in the

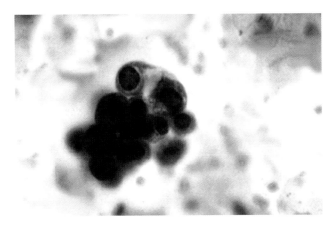

Fig. 5.12   Infarct. The cells exfoliating from an ischemic pulmonary parenchyma in a bronchial brush or an FNA can show marked nuclear atypia. However, poor preservation of cell membranes and a smudgy appearance of chromatin should alert to this possibility. (Papanicolaou, oil, ×100 objective). Slide from Ostrowski MO, Ramzy I, *In: Ramzy I: Clinical Cytopathology & Aspiration Biopsy, ed 2,* New York, NY, McGraw-Hill, 2000, with permission

early stages, a reflection of the hemorrhagic nature of pulmonary infarcts (Fig. 5.12). The number of atypical cells decreases in a few weeks and the background changes as healing progresses.

Key Features
- Atypical bronchial, squamous and alveolar cells as clusters
- Marked nuclear hyperchromasia
- Homogenization and clearing of chromatin
- Large nucleoli that maintain their round shape
- Ruptured cell walls and syncytial formation
- Hemorrhagic background and hemosiderin-laden macrophages

Differential diagnosis: Pulmonary infarcts can mimic adenocarcinoma in view of the degenerative cytoplasmic vacuoles associated with nuclear atypia. In other instances, the ischemic bronchial cells acquire cytoplasmic eosinophilia, and in the presence of nuclear atypia, may lead to the erroneous diagnosis of squamous cell carcinoma. However, the presence of only a few

atypical cells, degenerative nuclear features and chromatin smudging, and identification of cilia or terminal bars in the tight clusters
of bronchial cells distinguish ischemic changes from carcinoma.
Ischemic changes can be too bizarre to be true.

Suggested Reading

Aisner SC, Gupta PK, Frost JK. Sputum cytology in pulmonary sarcoidosis.
    Acta Cytol 1997;21:394–398
Dundore PA, Aisner SC, Templeton PA, et al. Nodular pulmonary amyloido-
    sis: diagnosis by fine-needle aspiration cytology and review of the litera-
    ture. Diagn Cytopathol 1993;9:562–564
Hsiu JG, Stitik FP, D'Amato NA, et al. Primary amyloidosis presenting as a
    unilateral hilar mass: report of a case by fine needle aspiration biopsy. Acta
    Cytol 1986;30:55–58
Silverman JF, Turner RC, West RL, et al. Bronchoalveolar lavage in the diag-
    nosis of lipoid pneumonia. Diagn Cytopathol 1989;5:3–8
Smojver-Jezek S, Peros-Golubicic T, Tekavec-Trkanjec J, et al. Trans-
    bronchial fine needle aspiration cytology in the diagnosis of mediasti-
    nal/hilar sarcoidosis. Cytopathology 2007;18:3–7
Sosolik RC, Gammon RR, Julius CJ, et al. Pulmonary alveolar proteinosis.
    A report of two cases with diagnostic features in bronchoalveolar lavage
    specimens. Acta Cytol 1998;42:377–383

Chapter 6
Benign Neoplasms

Benign neoplasms of lung are rare and cytologic samples are obtained usually by fine needle aspirations from mass lesions suspected of malignancy or an infectious disease, such as tuberculosis or fungal infections. The majority of the benign neoplasms have epithelial and mesenchymal components; pure benign epithelial neoplasms are extremely rare.

Pulmonary Hamartoma

Hamartomas occur more commonly in males with peak incidence in the 6th decade of life and present as well defined coin lesions in the lung and are usually correctly recognized by imaging techniques. In some instances, a suspicion of malignancy necessitates sampling by FNA. The material procured consists of epithelial cells, stromal elements and some lymphocytes (Figs. 6.1 and 6.2). The epithelial cells are bronchial type, with cilia or mucinous vacuoles, and appear singly or in sheets and strips, and have uniform nuclei. A variable amount of chondromyxoid stromal matrix and cells is seen. The myxoid component is fibrillary, interspersed with small spindled or oval cells. The cartilaginous fragments are usually thick, have sharply defined edges; they stain deep purple with the Diff-Quik and blue with Papanicolaou method (Figs. 6.3 and 6.4). Within the dark matrix, few lacunae containing chondrocytes

Y.S. Erozan, I. Ramzy, *Pulmonary Cytopathology*,
Essentials in Cytopathology 6, DOI 10.1007/978-0-387-88888-0_6,
© Springer Science+Business Media, LLC 2009

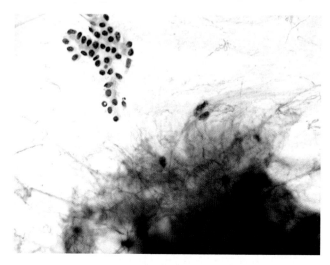

Fig. 6.1 Hamartoma. Myxoid and epithelial elements are seen in an FNA from a coin lesion in the left upper lobe (Papanicolaou, medium power)

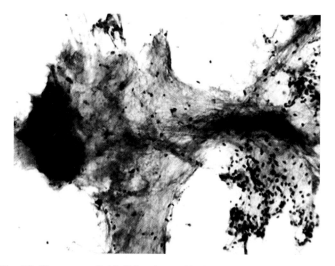

Fig. 6.2 Hamartoma. Epithelial and myxoid elements are evident in this air-dried FNA smear (Diff-Quik, low power)

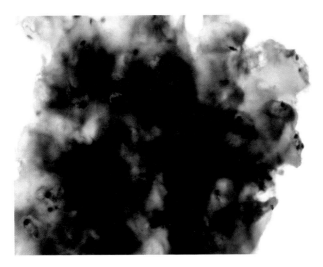

Fig. 6.3 Hamartoma. The cartilage fragment demonstrates sharp edges and a few chondrocytes (Papanicolaou, medium power)

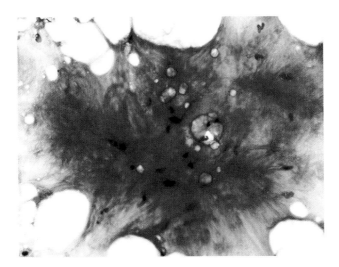

Fig. 6.4 Hamartoma. The matrix can be prominent when stained with a Romanowski type stain (Diff-Quik, medium power)

with yellowish brown cytoplasm and small nuclei can be identified. Respiratory epithelium may show reactive changes, and when it is the predominant component of the specimen, it may be mistaken for a well-differentiated adenocarcinoma. The presence of cilia and mesenchymal elements help to establish the correct diagnosis.

Key Features
- Sheets of bland ciliated and mucinous bronchial cells
- Fibrillary myxoid stroma with small uniform spindle cells
- Cartilaginous fragments, with sharply defined borders
- Chondrocytes in lacunae surrounded by dark purple matrix

Inflammatory Myofibroblastic Tumor

This benign neoplasm, previously referred to as inflammatory pseudotumor or plasma cell granuloma, is most probably of myofibroblastic derivation, as indicated by its immunohistochemical profile. FNA specimens are characterized by a mixture of bland fibroblasts and inflammatory cells that include lymphocytes, plasma cells, eosinophils and histiocytes. Reactive epithelial cells and entrapped bronchial cells are seen in the background. Necrosis and mitotic figures are lacking, and if present would indicate an aggressive fibrosarcoma. The spindle neoplastic cells are immunoreactive to vimentin, but not to cytokeratin, S-100 or CD34 (Fig. 6.5).

Key Features
- Bland spindled fibroblasts
- Infiltrate of lymphocytes, plasma cells, eosinophils and histiocytes
- Reactive bronchial epithelial cells
- Lacks necrosis or mitotic figures
- Spindle cells are vimentin positive, CK, CD 34 and S-100 negative

Differential diagnosis: Spindle cell carcinoma, malignant fibrous histiocytoma and pulmonary sarcomas are characterized by

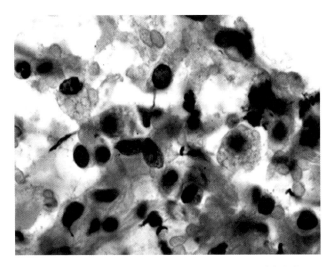

Fig. 6.5 Inflammatory myofibroblastic tumor. The FNA material depicts some oval or spindled cells. Careful correlation of the cytologic findings with of the clinical history and imaging studies is critical, in order to avoid misinterpretation of such cases (Papanicolaou, oil, ×100 objective)

nuclear pleomorphism, necrosis and active mitosis. In rare cases with predominantly histiocytic component, tightly packed histiocytes may mimic a non-small cell carcinoma (see "Non-small cell carcinoma, Differential diagnosis"). Immunohistochemistry is helpful, since the carcinoma will be cytokeratin positive and shows increased staining for p53. Malignant fibrous histiocytoma stains positively with histiocytic markers, including CD68 and α-1 antitrypsin. Bronchiolitis obliterans-organizing pneumonia (BOOP) is difficult to differentiate from inflammatory fibromyoblastic tumors since there is an overlap of clinical and cytologic features.

Solitary Fibrous Tumors

These are often small subpleural tumors that present as coin lesions or masses. Aspirates from these benign tumors are characterized by presence of monotonous spindle cells interspersed with variable amount of collagen fibers. Occasionally there is

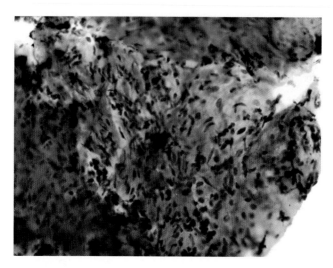

Fig. 6.6 Solitary fibrous tumor. A sheet of spindled stromal cells with fairly uniform nuclei is seen in this fine needle aspirate of a peripheral lung lesion (Papanicolaou, medium power)

significant nuclear atypia in the fibroblasts, and differentiation from true sarcomas becomes critical. Despite their nuclear atypia, solitary fibrous tumors lack necrosis or evidence of mitosis. Positive immunoreactivity to CD34 and lack of reactivity to cytokeratins help identify these neoplasms (Figs. 6.6 and 6.7A, B).

Key Features
- Subpleural well circumscribed mass
- Uniform spindle cells interspersed with mature collagen
- May show nuclear atypia
- Lacks necrosis and mitotic figures

Differential diagnosis: Malignant solitary fibrous tumors usually show evidence of increased mitotic activity as well as areas of necrosis. It is important to recognize that these features may be focal and not be represented in the sample, hence the importance of sampling more than one area of any large tumor if clinically feasible.

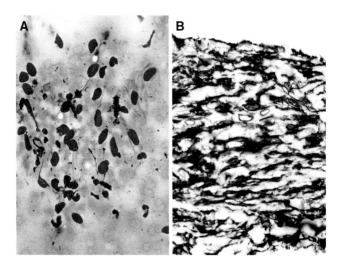

Fig. 6.7 Solitary fibrous tumor. (**A**) An air-dried preparation from the FNA shows abundant matrix, with a few spindled cells (Diff-Quik, high power). (**B**) Positive immunoreactivity with CD34 supports the diagnosis (CD34 Immunoperoxidase, diaminobenzidine (DAB) and hematoxylin, high power)

Pneumocytoma

This is a rare benign neoplasm of type II pneumocytes, usually encountered in middle-aged women as an incidental finding on chest radiographs. Most tumors are solitary and peripheral. The neoplasm was previously considered of endothelial origin (sclerosing hemangioma) because of some ultrastructural features and frequent association with hemorrhage. Immunohistochemical evidence, however, supports its origin from type II alveolar pneumocytes and Clara cells. The tumor is heterogeneous, with solid epithelioid, angiomatoid, sclerotic and papillary patterns. The neoplastic pneumocytes line septa that contain blood lakes, form papillary fronds or solid sheets surrounded by varying amounts of stroma. Gland-like structures may be seen entrapped within the sclerotic stroma. FNA results in hemorrhagic aspirates which may show papillae, solid sheets or isolated cells. The neoplastic cells are spindled or polygonal, with abundant pale eosinophilic cyto-

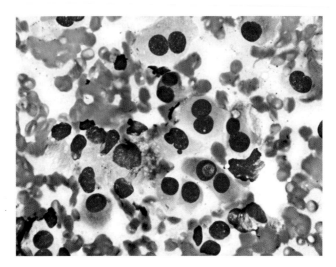

Fig. 6.8 Pneumocytoma. The aspirate is cellular, but the cells appear bland, and some have intranuclear cytoplasmic inclusions (Diff-Quik, oil, ×100 objective)

plasm that may be glycogen-rich (Fig. 6.8). The round to oval nuclei are quite bland, with fine evenly distributed chromatin and inconspicuous nucleoli. Intranuclear cytoplasmic inclusions are often seen (Fig. 6.9). The neoplastic cells are weakly positive for low molecular keratin, but strongly reactive to EMA and vimentin (Fig. 6.10). Additionally, they stain for surfactant and have osmophilic lamellar cytoplasmic bodies.

Key Features
- Most are incidental findings, usually in women
- Hemorrhagic aspirate
- Abundant polygonal type II pneumocytes and spindle cells
- Neoplastic cells arranged singly, in sheets or papillae
- Abundant eosinophilic cytoplasm, often glycogen-rich
- Nuclei oval, with bland evenly distributed chromatin
- Intranuclear cytoplasmic inclusions
- Cells weakly positive for low molecular weight keratin
- Strongly positive for EMA, vimentin and surfactant

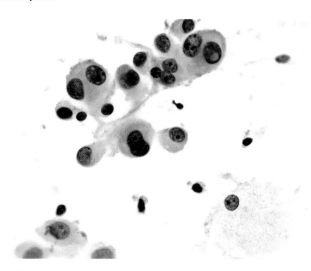

Fig. 6.9 Pneumocytoma. Note binucleation and the presence of intranuclear inclusions in some neoplastic cells. The nuclei are bland, unlike those of melanoma cells (Papanicolaou, oil, ×100 objective)

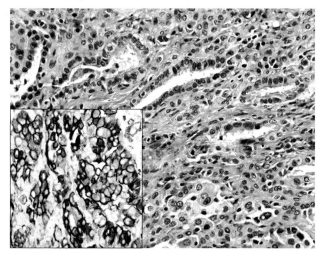

Fig. 6.10 Pneumocytoma. The histological section shows gland formation (H & E, medium power). *Inset* depicts immunoreactivity of the neoplastic cells to epithelial membrane antigen (EMA, Immunoperoxidase with diaminobenzidine (DAB) and hematoxylin, medium power)

Differential diagnosis: FNA of pneumocytoma can present a diagnostic challenge in differentiating it from bronchioloalveolar carcinoma, reactive pneumocytes and papillary neoplasms such as thyroid carcinoma and mesothelioma. Diagnostic bronchioloalveolar carcinoma cells have pleomorphic eccentric nuclei, thick nuclear membranes, coarser chromatin and prominent nucleoli. The cell groups have depth in focus and there is evidence of necrosis. Bronchioloalveolar carcinoma cells, however, may be bland similar to those of pneumocytoma, but the diagnosis of malignancy should not be established in the absence of unequivocal nuclear features to support that diagnosis, in view of the histologic and cytologic overlap between these two neoplasms (see Fig. 7.28). Reactive pneumocytes rarely appear in large numbers as seen with aspirates of pneumocytoma, and the clinical and imaging features do not indicate a well defined mass. Papillary thyroid carcinoma and mesothelioma show nuclear features of malignancy that differentiate them from the papillary fragments of pneumocytoma. Carcinoid tumors have monotonous uniform nuclei, but their chromatin is coarse "salt 'n pepper" like and the tumors are usually more centrally located. Immunostains can be helpful in differentiating pneumocytoma from all these tumors, but not from reactive pneumocytes.

Other Benign Tumors

Several, often microscopic, adenomas can be encountered in the lung periphery, but these are rarely aspirated. They include papillary Clara cell, bronchioloalveolar adenomas and clear cell adenomas. Differentiation of these tumors from pneumocytoma and reactive changes may be difficult and correlation with clinical and imaging features is critical. Bronchial granular cell tumors are rarely encountered in bronchial brushings or aspirates.

Suggested Reading

Ali SZ, Hoon V, Hoda S, et al. Solitary fibrous tumor. A cytologic-histologic study with clinical, radiologic, and immunohistochemical correlations. Cancer (Cancer Cytopathol) 1997;81:116–121

Armbruster C, Bernhardt K, Sertinek U. Pulmonary tumorlet: a case report of a diagnostic pitfall in cytology. Acta Cytol 2008;52:223–227

Bakhos, R, Wojcik EM, Olson MC. Transthoracic fine-needle aspiration cytology of inflammatory pseudotumor, fibrohistiocytic type: a case report with immunohistochemical studies. Diagn Cytopathol 1998;19:216–220

Baliga M, Flowers R, Heard K, et al. Solitary fibrous tumor of the lung: a case report with a study of the aspiration biopsy, histopathology, immunohistochemistry, and autopsy findings. Diagn Cytopathol 2007;35:239–244

Caruso RA, LaSpada F, Gaeta M, et al. Report of an intrapulmonary solitary fibrous tumor: fine-needle aspiration cytologic findings, clinicopathological, and immunohistochemical features. Diagn Cytopathol 1996;14:64–67

Chow LT, Chan SK, Chow WH, et al. Pulmonary sclerosing hemangioma. Report of a case with diagnosis by fine needle aspiration. Acta Cytol 1992;36:287–292

Hanna CD, Oliver DH, Liu J. Fine needle aspiration biopsy and immunostaining findings in an aggressive inflammatory myofibroblastic tumor of the lung. A case report. Acta Cytol 2007;51:239–246

Jin M-S, Ha H-J, Baek HJ, et al. Adenomyomatous hamartoma of lung mimicking benign mucinous tumor in fine needle aspiration biopsy: a case report. Acta Cytol 2008;52:357–360

Ramzy I. Pulmonary hamartomas: cytologic appearances of fine needle aspiratory biopsy. Acta Cytol 1976;20:15–19

Thunnissen FBMJ, Arends JW, Buchholtz RTF, et al. Fine needle aspiration cytology of inflammatory pseudotumor of the lung (plasma cell granuloma). Report of four cases. Acta Cytol 1989;33:917–921

Wang SE, Nieberg RK. Fine needle aspiration cytology of sclerosing hemangioma of the lung: a mimicker of bronchioloalveolar carcinoma. Acta Cytol 1986;30:51–54

Wiatrowska BA, Yazdi HM, Matzinger FR, et al. Fine needle aspiration biopsy of pulmonary hamartomas. Radiologic, cytologic and immunocytochemical study of 15 cases. Acta Cytol 1995;39:1167–1174

Wood B, Swarbrick N, Frost F. Diagnosis of pulmonary hamartoma by fine needle biopsy. Acta Cytol 2008;52:412–417

Zakharov V, Schinstine M. Hamartoma of the lung. Diagn Cytopathol 2008;36:331–332

Chapter 7
Primary Epithelial Malignancies

Lung cancer is the most common cancer in the world and is the leading cause of cancer deaths in both men and women in the United States. Almost all primary malignant neoplasms of lung (99.0%) are carcinomas. Four types: squamous cell carcinoma, adenocarcinoma, small cell carcinoma, and large cell carcinoma, constitute the majority of tumors. Carcinoid tumors, typical and atypical, comprise a small proportion of lung neoplasms. They belong to the category of neuroendocrine neoplasms which include large cell neuroendocrine carcinoma and small cell carcinoma; but they differ from the latter in regard to association with smoking, prognosis, and some other clinical aspects. Some lung carcinomas may have neuroendocrine differentiation demonstrated by immuno-histochemistry without the characteristic microscopic features of neuroendocrine differentiation. Although this could occur in all non-small cell carcinomas, it is most commonly seen in adenocar-cinomas. These tumors are reported according to their histological type with a note indicating the neuroendocrine differentiation.

Cytopathology plays an important role in the diagnosis of lung cancer as a non-invasive or minimally invasive diagnostic tech-nique. Definitive diagnosis of lung cancer can be established with high sensitivity and specificity. For practical purposes, lung carci-nomas are considered in two categories: small cell carcinoma and non-small cell carcinoma. Because of the differences in treatment and evaluation of prognosis, a differential diagnosis between these two categories is important and can be established by cytopathol-ogy with very high accuracy.

Y.S. Erozan, I. Ramzy, *Pulmonary Cytopathology*,
Essentials in Cytopathology 6, DOI 10.1007/978-0-387-88888-0_7,
© Springer Science+Business Media, LLC 2009

Squamous Cell Carcinoma

Squamous cell carcinoma is strongly related to cigarette smoking. It is the most common type of lung cancer among smokers, and over 90% of these tumors occur in smokers. The lesions include a spectrum of invasive carcinomas, which can be well differentiated or poorly differentiated, as well as preneoplastic changes in the form of dysplasia and carcinoma in situ. Although there is some overlap between the cytomorphologic features, careful assessment can be quite helpful in identifying the various components within this spectrum.

Well-Differentiated Squamous Cell Carcinomas

These tumors have predominantly keratinized tumor cells with markedly hyperchromatic nuclei with irregular borders. Keratinization is best seen in Papanicolaou-stained slides, and it typically has a dense, glassy appearance and deep orange (Halloween orange) color (Fig. 7.1), though the color may vary. Usually the entire cytoplasm is involved. Other forms are peripheral keratinization of the cytoplasm with non-keratinized center (endo-ectocytoplasm) (Fig. 7.2A) and Herxheimer spiral (Fig. 7.2B). Tumor cells tend to be single, especially in sputum, and commonly are seen in a necrotic background (Fig. 7.3). Small tissue fragments including pearl formations are present (Fig. 7.1). Intercellular bridges, another feature of squamous differentiation, are not commonly seen in cytologic samples. When present, they are usually found in fine-needle aspirations, or sometimes in bronchial brush material (Fig. 7.4A, B).

Key Features
- Predominantly single cells in sputum
- Hyperchromatic nuclei, some with sharp irregularities of nuclear borders
- Partially or diffusely keratinized cytoplasm
- Abnormal architecture (pearl formations) and shapes of cytoplasm (e.g., tadpole)
- Necrotic background

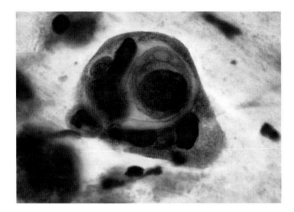

Fig. 7.1 Keratinizing squamous cell carcinoma. Transthoracic FNA. "Pearl" formation. The deep orange, glassy cytoplasm is typical of keratinization. Partial keratinization of cytoplasm, seen as the intracytoplasmic globules in one of the cells, represents an atypical form of keratinization. Such keratinization or pearl formation is not diagnostic for carcinoma without additional nuclear features of malignancy. (Papanicolaou stain, high power)

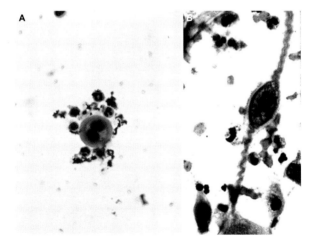

Fig. 7.2 Squamous cell carcinoma. Sputum. Atypical squamous differentiation. (**A**) Endo-ectocytoplasm. Note the dense, glassy ring at the periphery vs the lighter, delicate appearance of the cytoplasm around the nuclei. (**B**) Herxheimer spiral – bipolar tails of cytoplasm with a darker spiral in the center (Papanicolaou stain, high power)

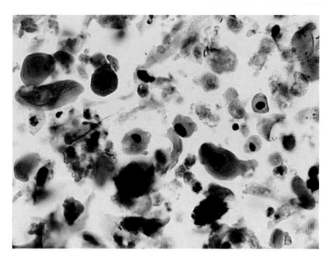

Fig. 7.3 Squamous cell carcinoma with necrotic changes. Transthoracic FNA. Note that most of the tumor cells show degenerative changes; only a few well-preserved cells establish the diagnosis (Papanicolaou stain, medium power)

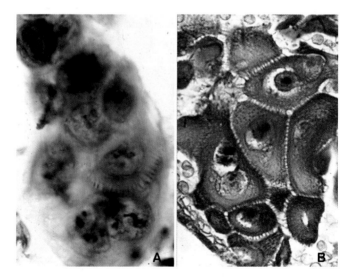

Fig. 7.4 Well differentiated squamous cell carcinoma. Transthoracic FNA. (**A, B**) Intercellular bridges. (**A**) Papanicolaou stain, high power. (**B**) Cell block, Hematoxylin and eosin stain, high power]

Poorly Differentiated Squamous Cell Carcinomas

These tumors tend to have more tissue fragments in cytologic samples. The majority of the cells have large nuclei with prominent nucleoli (Fig. 7.5). Hyperchromasia is less prominent than that found in well-differentiated squamous cell carcinomas. The presence of foci of squamous differentiation in some tissue fragments helps to determine the tumor type (Fig. 7.6). Most of these tumors, however, can only be diagnosed as poorly-differentiated non-small cell carcinoma.

Key Features
- Large nuclei
- Prominent nucleoli
- Occasional cells with squamous differentiation

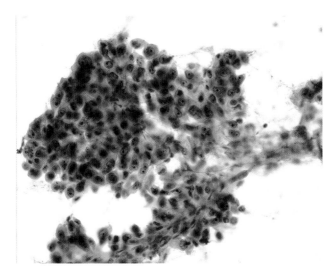

Fig. 7.5 Poorly differentiated squamous cell carcinoma. Transthoracic FNA. A large tissue fragment composed of tumor cells which have large nuclei with macronucleoli and varying nuclear/cytoplasmic ratios. No differentiation of cytoplasm is seen (Papanicolaou stain, medium power)

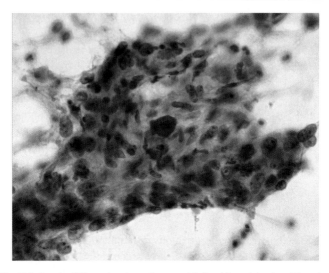

Fig. 7.6 Poorly differentiated carcinoma with focal keratinization. Transthoracic FNA (Papanicolaou stain, high power)

Immunohistochemistry

Most squamous cell carcinomas react to antibodies against high molecular weight cytokeratin (34BE12), cytokeratins 5/6, P63 and carcinoembryonic antigen (CEA). They are TTF-1 negative.

Differential Diagnosis of Invasive Squamous Cell Carcinoma

Certain benign conditions may be mistaken for squamous cell carcinoma (Table 7.1). Mistakes can be avoided by being aware of these conditions as well as the clinical history and radiological findings.

Table 7.1 Benign conditions mimicking squamous cell carcinoma

Epithelial atypias associated with:
    – Chemo/radio therapy
    – Viral infections
    – Inflammatory/reparative conditions
Artifacts (e.g., plant cells)

Chemotherapy and radiotherapy cause cellular atypia which may have some features of malignancy similar to poorly-differentiated non-small cell carcinomas. Typically, multiple or single enlarged nuclei with multiple prominent nucleoli, frayed cytoplasmic borders, and intracytoplasmic vacuoles are present (Fig. 7.7). The nuclei can be hyperchromatic, and irregular

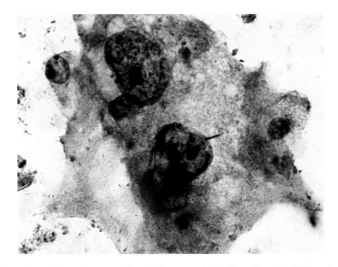

Fig. 7.7 Chemotherapy and radiotherapy effect. Transthoracic FNA. The patient had chemotherapy and radiotherapy for breast cancer. This fine needle aspirate is from a lung infiltrate which was thought to be lung cancer. Although there are markedly enlarged nuclei with macronucleoli, both nuclei and cytoplasm show markedly degenerative changes (Papanicolaou stain, high power)

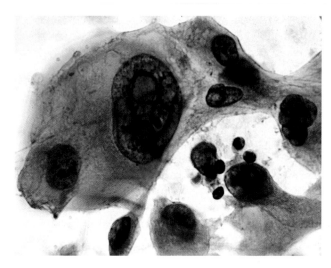

Fig. 7.8 Chemotherapy changes. A markedly atypical cell with intranuclear pseudoinclusion. Note the smudgy chromatin and intracytoplasmic vacuoles (Papanicolaou stain, high power)

clumping of chromatin may occur. Both nuclear and cyto-plasmic degenerative changes (e.g., blurry chromatin, intra-cytoplasmic vacuoles, loss of part of cytoplasm) are com-monly present. Rarely, intranuclear pseudoinclusions can be seen (Fig. 7.8).

Viral infections, specifically herpes, can have cellular changes which may be mistaken for malignancy when the typical fea-tures of viral infection (e.g., intranuclear inclusions) are not apparent (Fig. 7.9). By examining adequate samples, however, cells with characteristic features of herpes are usually found (Fig. 7.10). Caution should be used in diagnosing malignancy if the diagnosis is based on atypical cells with degenerative changes (Fig. 7.11).

Inflammatory and reparative conditions are common sources of false cancer diagnoses for both adenocarcinoma and squamous cell carcinomas. Atypical squamous metaplasia may occur in chronic inflammations associated with necrosis and cavity formation, such

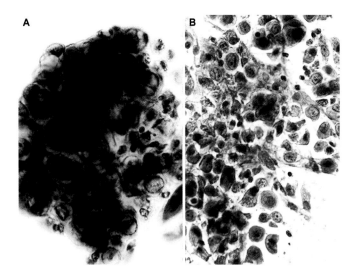

Fig. 7.9 Herpes simplex. Bronchial brush. Epithelial atypia mimicking poorly differentiated squamous cell carcinoma. Bronchial brush specimen. (**A**) Markedly enlarged, mostly hyperchromatic nuclei with high nuclear/cytoplasmic ratios in a thick tissue fragment. (**B**) Loosely arranged cells with large nuclei and prominent nucleoli. Note that some of the cells in (**A**) show gelatinous degeneration of chromatin, which should raise the suspicion of herpes infection (Papanicolaou stain, high power)

as bronchiectasis, abscess, and tuberculosis. A combination of atypical squamous cells and necrosis may mimic squamous cell carcinoma in FNAs and, rarely, in sputum specimens (Fig. 7.12. See also Figs. 4.1 and 4.2). Reparative processes occurring in the healing stages of pneumonia and pulmonary infarct are other sources of marked squamous atypia mimicking squamous cell carcinoma in FNA specimens.

Artifacts rarely cause a false cancer diagnosis. Nevertheless, some bizarre forms of plant cells resembling squamous cell carcinoma or poorly differentiated carcinomas can be found in sputum (Fig. 7.13A, B).

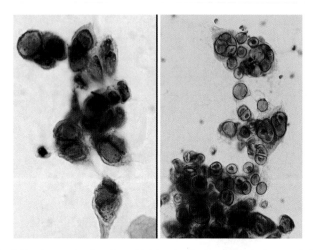

Fig. 7.10 Herpes simplex. Bronchial brush. Changes typical of herpes infection. (Repeat bronchial brush specimen from case shown in Fig. 7.9.) (Papanicolaou stain, high power)

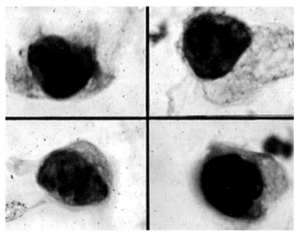

Fig. 7.11 Marked epithelial atypia mimicking poorly differentiated carcinoma. Sputum. Although the atypical cells have markedly enlarged, hyperchromatic nuclei, note the smudgy chromatin and vacuolated cytoplasm with frayed borders indicating degenerative changes. This patient had negative chest roentgenography, and no cancer developed during nine years of follow-up. No definitive cause of the changes was determined, but they are suspected to be due to a viral infection (Papanicolaou stain, high power)

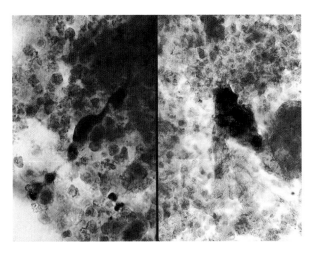

Fig. 7.12 Atypical squamous cells from cavitary tuberculosis. Transthoracic FNA. Fine needle aspiration of a cavitary lesion in the lung revealed these atypical squamous cells in a necrotic background. Ziehl-Neelson stain in this case revealed many acid-fast bacilli (Papanicolaou stain, high power)

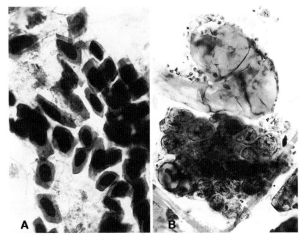

Fig. 7.13A,B Plant cells. Sputum. (**A**) The pinkish orangeophilic cytoplasm suggests keratinization, but it lacks the deep orange color and glassy appearance of cytoplasm. Furthermore, many of the cells have a rectangular or square shape, which is also consistent with plant cells. (**B**) These cells with large nuclei and high nuclear/cytoplasmic ratios resemble a poorly differentiated carcinoma. In other areas of the sputum, more typical plant cells were found. The patient did not have any malignancy (Papanicolaou stain, high power)

In Situ Squamous Cell Carcinoma and Dysplasia

Preinvasive stages of squamous cell carcinoma can be detected in sputum. Dysplasias and in situ carcinoma are often multifocal and early lesions tend to occur in segmental and subsegmental bronchi. Several large series reporting screening of populations at high risk for lung cancer (heavy smokers, uranium miners, tin miners) revealed the presence of atypical squamous cells in sputum before there was clinical or radiological evidence of lung cancer. The probability of lung cancer, present or future, correlated with the degree of squamous atypia.

Cytopathology of these lesions, presented below, is based on our observation of sputum samples obtained from asymptomatic smokers who participated in the "Cooperative Early Lung Cancer Detection Program" sponsored by the National Cancer Institute at the Johns Hopkins Medical Institutions, Mayo Clinic, and Memorial Hospital for Cancer.

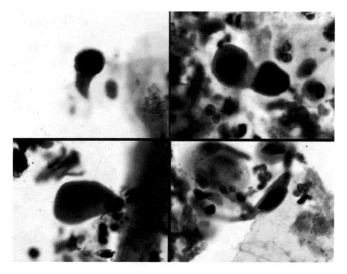

Fig. 7.14 Dysplasia (atypical metaplasia). Sputum. The cells shown are considered "moderate atypical metaplasia." Note the atypical cells which have enlarged nuclei with coarsely granular chromatin and keratinized cytoplasm. The cells may be round, polygonal, or atypically shaped (cytoplasmic tailing) (Papanicolaou stain, high power)

Cytopathology

Dysplasia (atypical metaplasia): In the "Early Lung Cancer Detection" project, the term "atypical metaplasia" is used. At Johns Hopkins, in the "ELC" protocol, atypical metaplasias are classified as slight (SAM), moderate (MAM), and grave (GAM). The degree of atypia is determined by nuclear changes (size, shape, irregularities of nuclear border, hyperchromasia) and nuclear cytoplasmic ratio. Examples of these are illustrated in (Fig. 7.14). The common features of dysplasia are hyperchromatic, usually round, nuclei with varying amounts of keratinized cytoplasm. Nucleoli are usually absent.

In situ squamous cell carcinoma: In sputum, the characteristic atypical cell population has round, hyperchromatic nuclei with scant keratinized cytoplasm (Fig. 7.15). However, large keratinized cells with apparent malignant features (Fig. 7.16) may

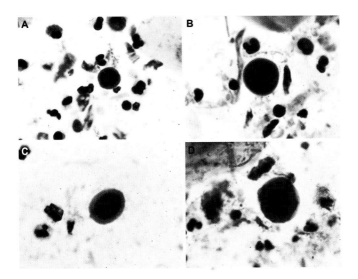

Fig. 7.15 In situ squamous cell carcinoma. Sputum. Note the small round cells with very scant keratinized cytoplasm (**A–C**). The cell shown in (**D**) has a large, hyperchromatic nucleus, but the larger cytoplasm is considered to be in the category of severe dysplasia (GAM) (Papanicolaou stain, high power)

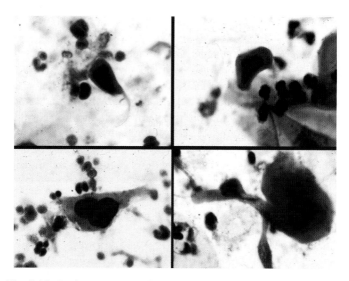

Fig. 7.16 In situ squamous cell carcinoma. Sputum. Neoplastic cells with hyperchromatic, round or irregularly shaped nuclei and pleomorphic cytoplasm. Identical cells would also be present in invasive squamous cell carcinoma (Papanicolaou stain, high power)

be seen. They are accompanied by a spectrum of atypical cells ranging from slight to marked atypia. The presence of nucleoli suggests a microinvasive or invasive carcinoma. The latter usually have a necrotic background, which is absent in both microinvasive and in situ squamous cell carcinoma. There is also an increased proportion of markedly atypical metaplastic squamous cells in microinvasive and invasive squamous cell carcinomas compared to in situ carcinoma. These features are summarized in Table 7.2.

Adenocarcinoma (Conventional and Bronchioloalveolar Types)

Adenocarcinomas are the most common type of lung cancer among women worldwide and, in men, exceed squamous cell carcinoma in certain countries (USA, Canada, China, and Japan).

Table 7.2 Cytomorphology of in situ, microinvasive and invasive squamous cell carcinoma

In situ carcinoma	Microinvasive carcinoma	Invasive carcinoma
Round keratinized cell with high n/c ratio and a spectrum of atypical metaplastic cells (SAM, MAM, GAM)	Cellular component similar to in situ except for larger proportion of GAM and cancer cells, and large keratinized cells with apparent nuclear atypia	Cellular component similar to microinvasive carcinoma
Large keratinized tumor cells with hyperchromatic nuclei may be present		
Nucleoli are absent	Nucleoli frequently present	Nucleoli are present in poorly differentiated squamous cell carcinoma
Necrosis is absent	Necrosis is absent	Necrosis is present

Adenocarcinomas, because of their peripheral locations, are asymptomatic in their early stages. They are usually detected by chest roentgenogram and diagnosed by transthoracic FNA. In advanced stages, with mediastinal, peribronchial/tracheal or carinal lymph node involvement, transbronchial/tracheal or EUS-guided (transesophageal) FNAs are used. Cells from adenocarcinoma are found in sputum usually in large tumors, mass lesions, or diffuse alveolar involvement, such as in bronchioloalveolar carcinoma.

Cytopathology of Conventional Adenocarcinoma

Well- and moderately-differentiated adenocarcinomas present predominantly tissue fragments. Evidence of glandular differentiation (i.e., luminal borders, partial or complete glandular structures) is present in some or most of the tissue fragments

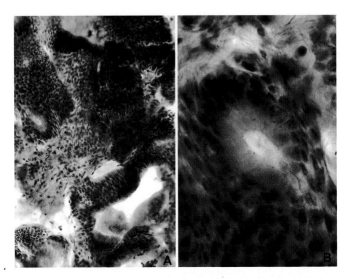

Fig. 7.17 Well differentiated adenocarcinoma. Thoracic FNA. (**A**) A large tissue fragment containing varying sized luminal spaces lined by well differentiated, tall columnar epithelium. Cellular atypia is minimal. (**B**) Basally-located, oval nuclei have a bland chromatin pattern and small nucleoli. Vertical orientation is preserved. The diagnosis of cancer is based on the abnormal architecture. [Papanicolaou stain; (**A**) low power, (**B**) high power]

(Figs. 7.17–7.19). Papillary formations may be present (Fig. 7.20). Nuclei are round or oval with rather bland, moderately increased chromatin and prominent, often single, nucleoli. Moderate amounts of delicate cytoplasm with distinct borders and sometimes with secretory vacuoles are characteristic features (Fig. 7.21). Some well-differentiated adenocarcinomas forming single layer tissue fragments may resemble benign respiratory epithelium; but even in the absence of the typical cellular features of malignancy, architectural abnormalities and variation in nuclear cytoplasmic relation among the cells forming the tissue fragments help to establish the diagnosis of malignancy. In adenocarcinomas, tumor cells in the fragment show significant variation in nuclear cytoplasmic ratio, location of the nucleus (peripheral vs central), and irregular

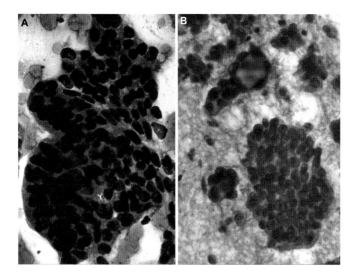

Fig. 7.18 Well differentiated adenocarcinoma. Transthoracic FNA. (**A**) Note the variation in size and shape of the enlarged nuclei and irregular distribution of the cells. Evidence of columnar (glandular) differentiation is seen at the periphery of the fragment. (**B**) Glandular formations and a hypercellular tissue fragment with luminal border. [(**A**) Diff-Quik stain, medium power, (**B**) Papanicolaou stain, medium power]

distribution of cells, unlike the regular "honey comb" pattern of benign columnar cells (Figs. 7.22 and 7.23).

Poorly differentiated adenocarcinomas also have predominantly tissue fragments, especially FNA specimens. Single tumor cells, however, are more often present than in well-differentiated tumors, and rarely may compose almost the entire cellular component in cytologic specimens. Cellular atypia is apparent with nuclear pleomorphism, varying (but usually high) nuclear cytoplasmic ratio, prominent nuclei, and marked architectural abnormalities. The presence of rare secretory vacuoles indicates the glandular differentiation in the tumor (Figs. 7.24 and 7.25). These tumors, in most cases, are classified as poorly-differentiated non-small cell carcinomas in limited cytologic or histologic specimens.

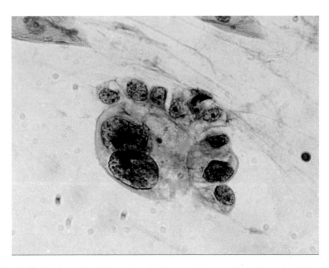

Fig. 7.19 Moderately differentiated adenocarcinoma. Transthoracic FNA. An abortive gland formation of atypical cells with large nuclei, prominent nucleoli, and delicate, vacuolated cytoplasm is seen (Papanicolaou stain, medium power)

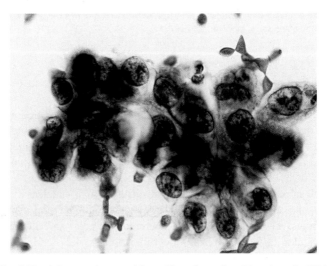

Fig. 7.20 Adenocarcinoma with papillary formation. Transthoracic FNA. Tumor cells have large, peripherally-located nuclei, macronucleoli, and delicate, vacuolated cytoplasm (Papanicolaou stain, medium power)

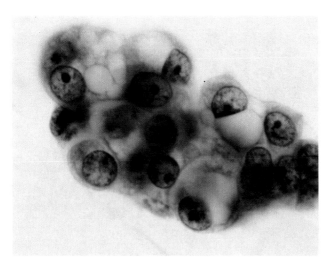

Fig. 7.21 Moderately differentiated adenocarcinoma. Transthoracic FNA. Note the large, round or ovoid nuclei with single macronucleoli, rather bland chromatin pattern, and delicate cytoplasm with single or multiple vacuoles (Papanicolaou stain, high power)

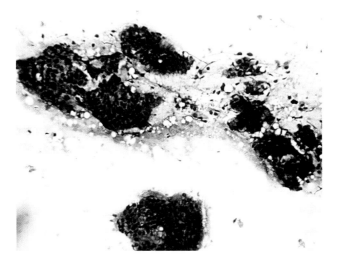

Fig. 7.22 Well differentiated mucinous adenocarcinoma. Transbronchial FNA. There are fragments of columnar-type epithelium which are difficult to distinguish from reactive respiratory epithelium with goblet cell hyperplasia on low power examination (Papanicolaou stain, low power)

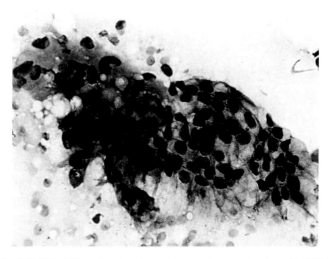

Fig. 7.23 Well differentiated mucinous adenocarcinoma. Transbronchial FNA. In the higher power view of one of the fragments shown in Fig. 7.22, variation in the nuclear size and shape as well as the amount of cytoplasm is apparent. Mucin-producing cells are mixed with foci of non-mucinous cells with higher nuclear/cytoplasmic ratio (Papanicolaou stain, high power)

Key Features
- Predominantly tissue fragments
- Disorganized cellular architecture in tissue fragments
- Variation in nuclear cytoplasmic relation (n/c ratio, location of nucleus) among cells in a tissue fragment
- Enlarged nuclei with prominent nucleoli
- Intracytoplasmic vacuoles
- Poorly differentiated adenocarcinomas may have predominantly single cells

Cytopathology of Bronchioloalveolar Carcinoma

Bronchioloalveolar carcinomas (BAC) may appear in monolayer tissue fragments, smaller tissue fragments with undulated borders, or single cells with mucin vacuoles. The latter are more commonly seen in sputum (Fig. 7.26). The non-mucinous type BAC may

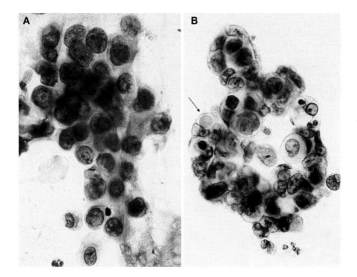

Fig. 7.24 Poorly differentiated adenocarcinoma. Transthoracic FNA. (**A**) An aggregate of tumor cells with large nuclei, prominent nucleoli, and high nuclear/cytoplasmic ratio. No evidence of glandular differentiation is present. (**B**) A tissue fragment of tumor with large pleomorphic nuclei and varying amounts of cytoplasm. Scattered large intracytoplasmic vacuoles, one containing globular secretory material (*arrow*), indicate the glandular differentiation (Papanicolaou stain, high power)

show papillary formations (Fig. 7.27). Monolayer tissue fragments usually occur in transthoracic FNA specimens (Fig. 7.28). Nuclei of BAC are usually round and uniform with vesicular chromatin and small nucleoli.

Most adenocarcinomas are histologically mixed subtypes and may have a BAC component. Those are reported as adenocarcinoma with bronchioloalveolar features (Fig. 7.29).

Immunohistochemistry of Adenocarcinomas

Adenocarcinomas express epithelial antigens, AE1/AE3, epithelial membrane antigen (EMA), CAM 5.2, and carcinoembryonic

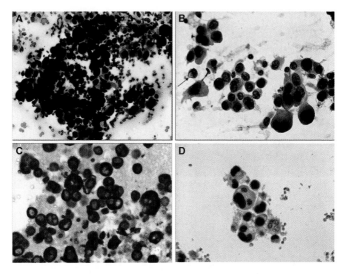

Fig. 7.25 Poorly differentiated adenocarcinoma. Transthoracic FNA. (**A**) Predominantly single tumor cells with large nuclei and varying amounts of cytoplasm. This cytomorphology is not different from that of large cell carcinoma. (**B**) Tumor cells similar to those in (**A**). The presence of an intracytoplasmic vacuole with globular, secretory material (*arrow*) indicates glandular differentiation. (**C**) Immunostain for CK7 and (**D**) immunostain for TTF-1 are strongly positive. [(**A**) Diff-Quik stain, medium power; (**B**) Papanicolaou stain, high power; (**C&D**) high power]

antigen. TTF-1 is usually positive. They are more frequently positive for CK7 than CK20 (Fig. 7.25 C, D). Mucinous tumors, especially mucinous BAC, do not react to immunostains for TTF-1, and they are frequently positive for CK20 as well as CK7.

Key features of mucinous bronchioloalveolar carcinoma

- Predominantly single cells and small tissue fragments in sputum and BAL
- Monolayer tissue fragments in FNA specimens
- Cytoplasmic large vacuoles
- Uniform, round nuclei with bland chromatin pattern and prominent nucleoli

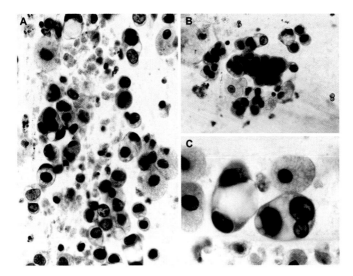

Fig. 7.26 Bronchioloalveolar carcinoma, mucinous type. Sputum. (**A**) Predominantly single cells and rare small tissue fragments. Enlarged hyperchromatic nuclei and large, intracytoplasmic vacuoles are seen in some of the cells. (**B**) Several tissue fragments which are composed of relatively small cells with scant cytoplasm, some containing small vacuoles. (**C**) A group of tumor cells with varying morphology. Note a hyperdistended vacuole between two cells, one of the characteristic features of mucinous bronchioloalveolar carcinoma in sputum. [Papanicolaou stain; (**A**, **B**) medium power, (**C**) high power]

Key features of nonmucinous bronchioloalveolar carcinoma
- Tissue fragments, some in papillary forms
- Small tissue fragments with undulated borders (hobnail appearance)
- Round, uniform nuclei with bland chromatin pattern
- Scant cytoplasm

Differential Diagnosis of Adenocarcinomas

A variety of benign and malignant conditions may have similar morphology to that of primary adenocarcinoma, both the conventional and bronchioloalveolar types. Emphasis here is given to

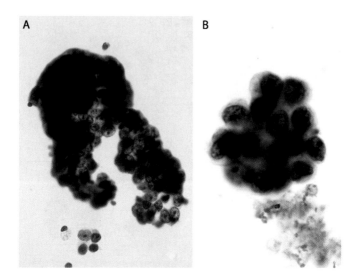

Fig. 7.27 Bronchioloalveolar carcinoma, non-mucinous type. **A**) Bronchial wash. A hypercellular, papillary-like tissue fragment composed of tumor cells with monotonous morphology. Tumor cells display round or ovoid nuclei with vesicular chromatin and prominent nucleoli. Note the sharply defined "luminal border" formation at the periphery of the upper part of the fragment. (**B**) Transthoracic FNA. Another tissue fragment of BAC. In contrast to that in (**A**), this has an undulated border formed by loosely attached cells with coarsely granular chromatin and somewhat irregular nuclear borders. Similar arrangements of cells also occur in reactive alveolar cell hyperplasia. Although the overall appearance (i.e., high nuclear/cytoplasmic ratio, nuclear border irregularities along with single prominent nucleoli) is more consistent with a malignant neoplasm, definitive diagnosis should be made cautiously if only a few of these fragments are present (Papanicolaou stain, high power, oil, ×100 objective)

common diagnostic problems, but some rare conditions we have seen in our practice are also included.

Benign conditions mimicking adenocarcinoma: These conditions are listed in Table 7.3. Reactive changes in the respiratory epithelium of the tracheobronchial tree and alveolar cell proliferation in response to injury are the most common conditions which may have some features similar to adenocarcinoma. The causes of

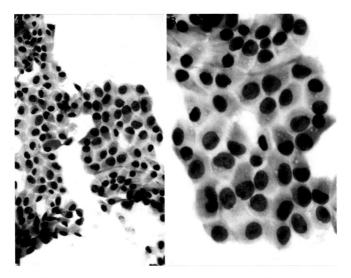

Fig. 7.28 Bronchioloalveolar carcinoma. Transthoracic FNA. (**A**) Monolayer sheets of loosely arranged cells which have large, eccentrically located, round or ovoid nuclei with bland chromatin patterns. Small nucleoli and slight irregularity of the nuclear borders are seen in some of the cells under high power. (**B**) The majority of the tumor cells have moderate amounts of cytoplasm and vary in shape, but are mostly polygonal or columnar, with indistinct borders. There is a resemblance to the sheet of mesothelial cells sometimes seen in transthoracic FNAs, but those usually have centrally located nuclei and dense cytoplasm with distinct borders (see Fig. 7.44 (A). [Papanicolaou stain; (**A**) medium power, (**B**) high power]

these changes include infections (especially viral), irritants (e.g., tobacco smoke, asbestos) and some chemicals.

Fragments of respiratory epithelium with varying degrees of atypia can be seen in viral infections, asthma or allergic bronchitis, hamartoma, and on rare occasions, pulmonary sequestration, inflammatory myofibroblastic tumor and lipid pneumonia. *Viral infections,* especially herpes, can cause significant atypia which may be mistaken for a poorly differentiated carcinoma if the characteristic viral changes are not evident. In sputum specimens from patients with asthma or allergic bronchitis, fragments of hypersecretory respiratory epithelium (Creola bodies)

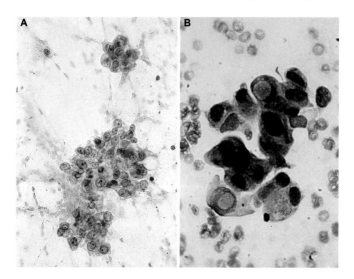

Fig. 7.29 Adenocarcinoma with bronchioloalveolar features. Transthoracic FNA. (**A**) The arrangement of the cells, as well as the individual cell morphology, are similar to those seen in BAC, but they can also be present in well differentiated adenocarcinomas. (**B**) Intranuclear cytoplasmic inclusions are more commonly seen in BAC than in conventional adenocarcinomas. [(**A**) Papanicolaou stain, medium power. (**B**) Diff-Quik stain, high power]

with enlarged nuclei and prominent nucleoli may mimic adenocarcinoma (Fig. 7.30A, B). The presence of cilia indicates the benign nature of these epithelial fragments. In addition, esoinophils and Curschmann spirals may be present and support this diagnosis (See Chapter 3).

Table 7.3 Benign conditions mimicking adenocarcinoma

Proliferative/reactive changes
  – Respiratory epithelium (trachea, bronchi)
  – Atypical alveolar proliferation
Hamartoma (respiratory epithelium)
Pulmonary sequestration (respiratory epithelium)
Inflammatory pseudotumor (epithelioid histiocytes)

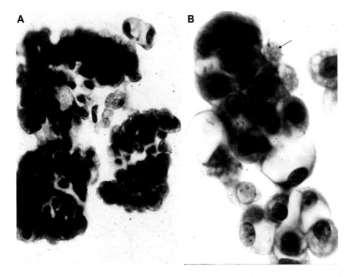

Fig. 7.30 Reactive hypersecretory respiratory epithelium (Creola bodies). Sputum. Fragments of reactive respiratory epithelium with enlarged nuclei and large mucus vacuoles. (**A**) Most fragments display apparent cilia. (**B**) Enlarged nuclei with prominent nucleoli and large, single, cytoplasmic vacuoles suggest an adenocarcinoma, but the presence of terminal plates with cilia (*arrow*) indicates the benign nature of the changes. [Papanicolaou stain; (**A**) low power, (**B**) high power]

Hamartoma is another source of respiratory epithelial fragments which may be found in abundance in fine needle aspirations and cause false diagnosis or suspicion of adenocarcinoma (Fig. 7.31A). Again, the presence of cilia, mesenchymal myxofibroid, or cartilaginous tissue is helpful in the differential diagnosis (See Chapter 3). In some cases with limited sampling, however, nonepithelial elements of hamartoma may not be present and reactive epithelium may exhibit significant atypia (Fig. 7.31B, C). An unusual case of hamartoma mimicking metastatic carcinoma of breast is shown in Fig. 7.32A, D. In most cases, radiological and clinical correlations help to establish the diagnosis.

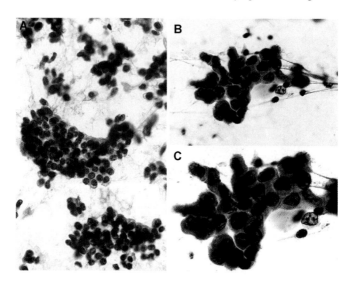

Fig. 7.31 Hamartoma. Fragments of respiratory epithelium. Transthoracic FNA. (**A**) Many fragments of respiratory epithelium are present, but without cartilaginous or mesenchymal tissue. Note the cilia in several tissue fragments and single cells. (**B**, **C**) Reactive respiratory epithelium with marked atypia. There are enlarged nuclei with prominent nucleoli and some with sharp irregularities of the nuclear envelope. The cells have varying amounts of cytoplasm and generally high nuclear/cytoplasmic ratios. The normal architecture is disturbed. In this case, malignancy cannot be ruled out. [Papanicolaou stain; (**A**) low power, (**B**) medium power, (**C**) high power]

Pulmonary sequestration is a rare condition which may present as a mass lesion radiologically suspicious for malignancy. Because of the enlarged respiratory spaces, needle aspirations contain large tissue fragments which should be differentiated from a well-differentiated adenocarcinoma (Fig. 7.33A–C). They lack the architectural abnormalities described in the well differentiated adenocarcinomas.

In *lipid pneumonia*, macrophages with enlarged nuclei, prominent nucleoli, and large cytoplasmic fat vacuoles may mimic adenocarcinoma in sputum and BAL specimens. Oil Red O stain demonstrates the cytoplasmic lipid (Fig. 7.34).

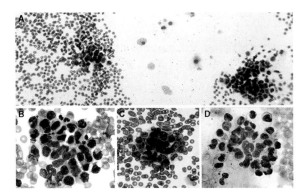

Fig. 7.32 Hamartoma. Transthoracic FNA from a single nodule in a patient with a history of lobular carcinoma of breast. (**A**) Only these three tight clusters of atypical cells were found in the specimen. (**B–D**) Cells have enlarged nuclei, which vary in size and shape, and ill defined cytoplasm. Based on these features and the clinical history, they were thought to represent a metastatic breast carcinoma. Wedge resection of the lesion revealed hamartoma. [Diff-Quik stain; (**A**) low power (**B–D**) high power]

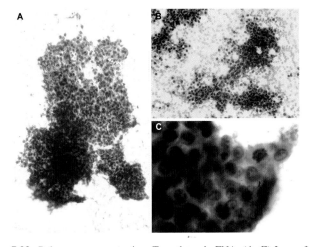

Fig. 7.33 Pulmonary sequestration. Transthoracic FNA. (**A–C**) Large fragments of columnar epithelium. One area of reactive epithelium with enlarged nuclei and a mitosis is shown in (**C**). [(**A, C**) Papanicolaou stain, (**B**) Diff-Quik stain; (**A, B**) low power, (**C**) high power]

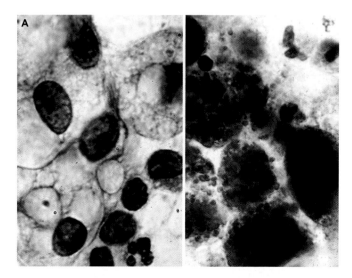

Fig. 7.34 Lipid pneumonia. Sputum. (**A**) Macrophages with enlarged nuclei (compare with the size of the neutrophil at the lower edge of the picture), prominent nucleoli, and large cytoplasmic vacuoles mimicking adenocarcinoma. (**B**) Positive staining with Oil red O. [(**A**) Papanicolaou stain, (**B**) Oil red O stain, (**A&B**) High power, oil, ×100 objective]

Fine needle aspirates of *inflammatory myofibroblastic tumor,* in rare instances, may be composed almost entirely of tightly packed histiocytes (epithelioid histiocytes) which mimic a poorly-differentiated non-small cell carcinoma (Fig. 7.35). Intranuclear cytoplasmic inclusions may be seen (Fig. 7.36). Immunostains for epithelia and macrophages might be necessary to make a definitive differential diagnosis.

Large Cell Carcinoma (LCC)

This is an undifferentiated non-small cell carcinoma which lacks the features of squamous or glandular differentiation. It is

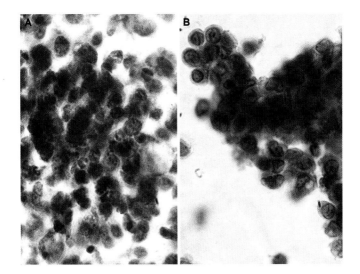

Fig. 7.35 Inflammatory myofibroblastic tumor. Transthoracic FNA. (**A**, **B**) Tightly packed cells with large nuclei and scant to moderate amounts of cytoplasm displaying an epithelial-like arrangement. Nuclear border irregularities (i.e., irregular thickening and sharp indentations of the nuclear envelope), which are more prominent in (**B**), appear to represent degenerative changes along with other features of degeneration such as blurry chromatin, ill defined cytoplasmic borders, and vacuolation of cytoplasm. [(**A**) Papanicolaou stain; (**B**) Hematoxylin and eosin; high power]

diagnosed by exclusion. Specificity of this type in limited samples, such as FNAs of small biopsies, is low. Therefore, they are generally reported in the broad category of "poorly-differentiated non-small cell carcinoma" and comprise about 9% of lung cancers. Most of these tumors occur in male smokers and are localized peripherally.

A subtype of LCC, large cell neuroendocrine carcinoma (LCNEC), comprises about 3% of lung cancers. Other rare subtypes are basoloid carcinoma, lymphoepithelioma-like carcinoma, clear cell carcinoma and large cell carcinoma with rhabdoid phenotype. These rare subtypes, with the exception of lymphoepithelioma-like carcinoma, are all associated with

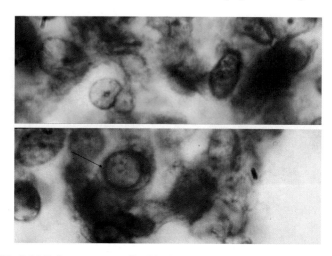

Fig. 7.36 Inflammatory myofibroblastic tumor. Transthoracic FNA. Intranuclear cytoplasmic inclusions (Papanicolaou stain, high power oil, ×100 objective)

smoking. These will not be discussed separately, but will be referred to in the differential diagnosis where indicated.

Cytopathology of Large Cell Carcinomas

Fine needle aspirates of large cell carcinomas are usually cellular and contain single cells and tissue fragments of undifferentiated tumor cells which have large nuclei with moderate amounts of cytoplasm with increased n/c ratio. Neoplastic cells display a varying degree of nuclear pleomorphism with single or multiple, large nucleoli (Fig. 7.37A, B). Multinucleated tumor giant cells may be present (Fig. 7.38A, B).

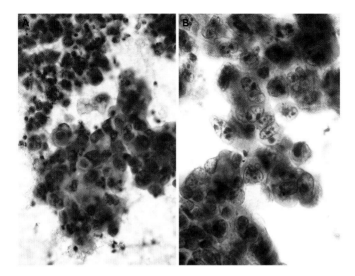

Fig. 7.37 Large cell carcinoma. Transthoracic FNA. (**A**) A tissue fragment composed of disorganized large tumor cells with pleomorphic nuclei. (**B**) Large undifferentiated tumor cells with pleomorphic nuclei and macronucle-oli. [Papanicolaou stain. (**A**) medium power, (**B**) high power]

Large cell neuroendocrine carcinomas show nuclear molding, palisading, and rosette formations similar to other neuroendocrine tumors, but they are composed of larger cells than those of small cell carcinoma and have prominent nucleoli. In small samples, these features may not be apparent. Immunoperoxidase stains with antibodies to neuroendocrine cellular component are necessary to establish the specific diagnosis (Fig. 7.39A, B).

Key features: large cell carcinoma (LCC)
- Tumor cell with large nuclei and prominent nucleoli
- Absence of glandular or squamous differentiation
- Necrosis and mitoses are common

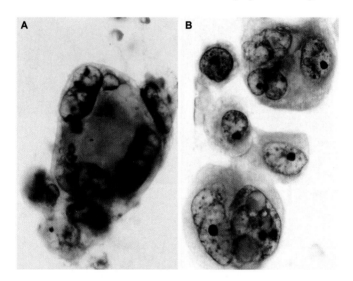

Fig. 7.38 Large cell carcinoma. Transthoracic FNA. (**A**) A multinucleated neoplastic giant cell. Marked variation in nuclear size and irregular chromatin clumping are features of malignancy. (**B**) Multinucleated neoplastic cells exhibiting pleomorphic nuclei and macronucleoli (Papanicolaou stain, high power, oil, ×100 objective)

Key features: large cell neuroendocrine carcinoma (LCNEC)

- Tumor cell with neuroendocrine features
- Prominent nucleoli
- Necrosis

Differential Diagnosis

Large cell carcinoma (NOS) should be differentiated from neuroendocrine large cell carcinoma, poorly-differentiated squamous and adenocarcinomas, other metastatic poorly-differentiated carcinomas or sarcomas, and anaplastic lymphoma. Positive staining with neuroendocrine markers of LCNEC differentiates it from LCC (Fig. 7.39B). LCNEC is differentiated from small cell carcinoma by having larger nuclei and prominent nucleoli. Positive staining with neuroendocrine markers differentiates it from

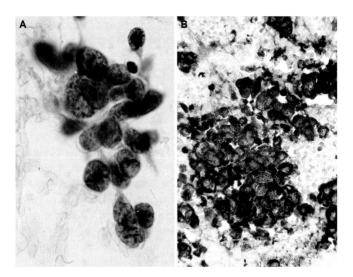

Fig. 7.39 Large cell neuroendocrine carcinoma. Transthoracic FNA. (**A**) Large neoplastic cells displaying round, oval or irregularly shaped nuclei, ill-defined cytoplasm and focal nuclear molding. Nuclei have coarse chromatin patterns with chromocenter. (**B**) Immunoperoxidase stain for chromogranin is strongly positive. [(**A**) Papanicolaou stain, high power; (**B**) Immunoperoxidase stain for chromogranin, medium power]

basaloid carcinomas which also show peripheral palisading of cells in larger tissue fragments in fine needle aspirates. Differential diagnosis among the types of poorly-differentiated non-small cell carcinomas (PDNSC) is usually difficult in both cytologic samples and small biopsies, such as core needle biopsies. In some, focal evidence of glandular or squamous differentiation can be found. Mucin stains are helpful in differentiating LCC from poorly differentiated adenocarcinoma.

Small Cell Carcinoma

Small cell carcinomas comprise 20% of lung cancers and, like squamous cell carcinomas, are strongly associated with smoking.

At the time of diagnosis, they usually present as a large hilar mass. The microscopic diagnosis is established by bronchoscopic cytologic (transbronchial/tracheal FNA) or histologic samples. Sputum specimens can also provide the diagnosis, but with lesser sensitivity compared to the yield for squamous cell carcinoma. Rare peripheral small cell carcinomas are diagnosed by percutaneous (transthoracic) FNA.

In the current WHO classification, small cell carcinomas are divided into two categories: small cell carcinoma and combined small cell carcinoma. *Small cell carcinoma* is defined as a malignant neoplasm composed of small cells with scant cytoplasm, finely granular, evenly dispersed chromatin, absent or inconspicuous nucleoli, and prominent nuclear molding. *Combined small cell carcinoma* has an additional component consisting of any of the types of non-small cell carcinoma, usually adenocarcinoma, squamous cell carcinoma, or large cell carcinoma.

Cytopathology of Small Cell Carcinoma

Cellularity and presentation of tumor (single cells, groups, tissue fragments, etc.) vary according to the collection technique. In sputum specimens, tumor cells appear as single cells, small groups, and linear forms in mucus strands and are commonly associated with a necrotic background (Figs. 7.40 and 7.41). Bronchoscopic brush specimens have more tissue fragments than sputum. Columns of molded tumor cells, once referred to as "vertebralike" formations, can be seen (Fig. 7.42A). FNAs, both transthoracic and transbronchial, yield varying proportions of single cells and tissue fragments associated with necrotic debris and apoptotic bodies (Figs. 7.42B, 7.43–7.46). Tumor cells range from slightly larger than small lymphocytes ("oat cell type") to about three times the size of the mature lymphocyte with scant, ill-defined cytoplasm. Nuclei can be round, oval or spindle shaped, and in well-preserved tumor cells have evenly dispersed granular chromatin pattern, but less preserved cells may have diffuse hyperchromasia. Nucleoli are absent or inconspicuous. Nuclear molding is

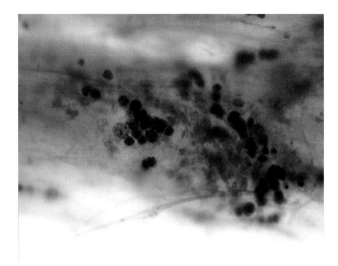

Fig. 7.40 Small cell carcinoma. Sputum. Neoplastic cells displaying hyper-chromatic, round or irregularly shaped nuclei forming columns with nuclear molding in the necrotic background (Papanicolaou stain, medium power)

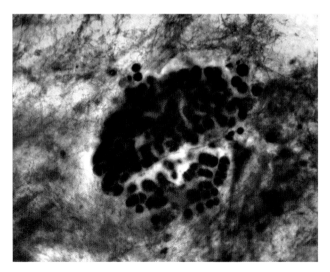

Fig. 7.41 Small cell carcinoma. Sputum. Larger tissue fragments, columns, and single cell forms of the neoplasm in a necrotic background. (Papanicolaou stain, high power)

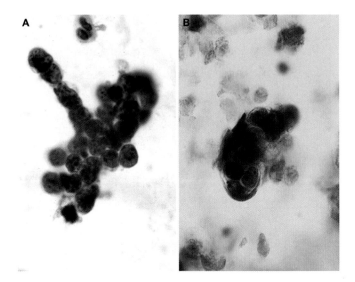

Fig. 7.42 Small cell carcinoma. (**A**) Bronchial brush. Columnar formations (vertebra-like) with nuclear molding. (**B**) Transthoracic FNA. A tissue fragment composed of neoplastic cells tightly wrapped around each other in a necrotic background. This is more commonly seen in effusions and is referred to as an "onion skin-like" formation. The cells have extremely high nuclear/cytoplasmic ratios and display cytoplasm to nuclear molding (Papanicolaou stain, high power)

actually molding of the cytoplasm of one tumor cell to the other cell's nucleus changing the shape of the latter, as seen in well-preserved cells (Fig. 7.42B).

Immunocytochemistry: Small cell carcinomas react to antibodies for CD56, synaptophysin, chromogranin, TTF-1, and CEA.

Key Features
- Small cells with high n/c ratio
- No prominent nucleoli
- Nuclear molding
- Mitoses
- Necrotic background

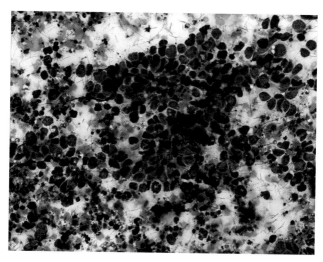

Fig. 7.43 Small cell carcinoma. Transbronchial FNA. Note the nuclear molding, mitotic figures, and necrotic background with apoptotic bodies (Diff-Quik stain, high power)

Differential diagnosis: The majority of small cell carcinomas with typical morphology are diagnosed without difficulty. Some benign conditions and malignant neoplasms, however, may be mistaken for small cell carcinomas (Table 7.4). In bronchial brush specimens, hyperplastic reserve cells appear in forms of varying sized tissue fragments or small groups and single cells, and may not have attached ciliated columnar epithelium. Although they have high nuclear cytoplasmic ratio, nuclear molding is not present. In air-dried or poorly alcohol fixed preparations, nuclei of reserve cells and degenerated columnar cells may mimic small cell carcinoma displaying nuclear molding (Fig. 7.47). Aggregates of lymphocytes in transbronchial FNAs may give the appearance of nuclear molding on air-dried, Diff-Quik stained slides, raising the suspicion of small cell carcinoma. In alcohol fixed slides, however, the single cell pattern is apparent.

Other malignant neoplasms which may mimic small cell carcinoma are shown on Table 7.4. Differential diagnosis between

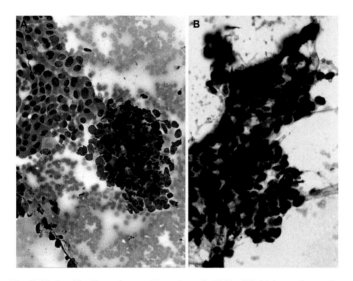

Fig. 7.44 Small cell carcinoma. Transthoracic FNA. (**A**) A sheet of mesothe-lial cells and a tight cluster of small neoplastic cells with round or ovoid nuclei and indistinct cytoplasm. (**B**) A hypercellular tissue fragment composed of disorganized neoplastic cells with hyperchromatic ovoid nuclei and indis-tinct cytoplasm. [(**A**) Diff-Quik stain, (**B**) Papanicolaou stain, (**A&B**) medium power]

a small cell carcinoma and poorly-differentiated non-small cell carcinomas can be challenging when the former is composed of somewhat larger cells. The majority of poorly differentiated carcinomas have prominent nucleoli and larger cytoplasm. The most reliable diagnostic features of small cell carcinoma are very high nuclear cytoplasmic ratio and absence of prominent nucleoli (Fig. 7.48A&B). Immunostains for p63 and TTF-1 are helpful in the differential diagnosis between poorly differenti-ated squamous cell carcinoma and small cell carcinoma. The former reacts to immunostain for p63, but it does not react to the stain for TTF-1. Reactions to these stains are reversed in small cell carcinoma. Rare cases of basaloid carcinoma, primary or metastatic, would be very difficult, if not impossible, to dif-ferentiate from small cell carcinoma by cytomorphology alone

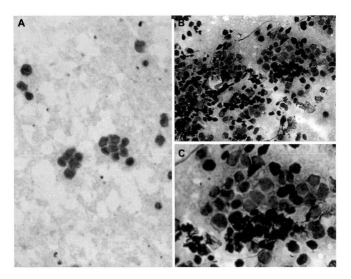

Fig. 7.45 Small cell carcinoma. Transbronchial FNA. Neoplastic cells mixed with lymphocytes. The former display nuclear molding, which is more apparent in (**A**), and they are larger than the lymphocytes in (B, C). [(**A**) Papanicolaou stain, medium power, (**B**) Diff-Quik stain, medium power, (**C**) Diff-Quik stain, high power]

(Fig. 7.49). These tumors, however, do not express TTF-1 and generally do not react to neuroendocrine markers. Lymphomas differ from small cell carcinomas by their single cell appearance (Fig. 7.50A, B). Phenotyping studies using flow cytometry and/or immunostaining for lymphoid markers may be needed in borderline cases. Among other neuroendocrine tumors, carcinoid tumor and metastatic Merkel cell carcinoma can be difficult to differentiate from small cell carcinoma. Carcinoid tumors lack the necrotic background, usually have more cytoplasm, and tissue fragments may show nuclear overlapping, but usually not nuclear molding. They also lack the necrotic background and mitoses. Merkel cell carcinoma has a similar cytomorphology to small cell carcinoma but differs from the latter with positive staining with CK20, but not with CK7 and TTF1.

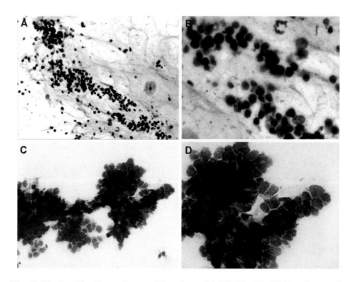

Fig. 7.46 Small cell carcinoma. Transbronchial FNA. (**A**, **B**) Small, mostly single neoplastic cells mixed with lymphocytes. A definitive diagnosis of small cell carcinoma cannot be made based on these cells alone. (**C**, **D**) A tissue fragment of the neoplasm from the same specimen exhibiting the characteristic features of small cell carcinoma. [(**A,B**) Papanicolaou stain; (**A**) low power, (**B**) high power; (**C**, **D**) Diff-Quik stain, (**C**) medium power, (**D**) high power]

Table 7.4 Conditions mimicking small cell carcinoma

Benign conditions
Reserve cell hyperplasia
Lymphoid hyperplasia
Malignant neoplasms
Lymphomas/leukemias
Poorly differentiated carcinomas
Carcinoid tumor
Metastatic carcinomas (e.g., Merkel cell, breast and endometrial carcinomas)

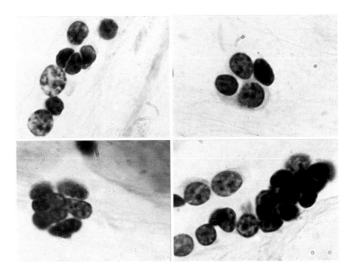

Fig. 7.47 Poorly preserved columnar epithelium and reserve cells mimicking small cell carcinoma. Bronchial/brush/wash. Mostly bare nuclei, only a few cells with partially preserved ill-defined cytoplasm, indicative of degenerative changes. The nuclei also exhibit degenerative changes, such as blurry chromatin. The focal nuclear molding seen here should be interpreted cautiously as evidence of small cell carcinoma (Papanicolaou stain, high power)

Neuroendocrine Neoplasms

This subset of lung tumors, which includes typical and atypical carcinoid, large cell neuroendocrine carcinoma and small cell carcinoma, react to one or more neuroendocrine markers (i.e., CD56, chromogranin, synaptophysin) and have some common architectural patterns, such as organized nesting, palisading, trabecular pattern and rosette-like structures. High-grade neuroendocrine neoplasms, small cell carcinoma and large cell neuroendocrine carcinoma have been discussed previously under the four major categories of primary lung carcinoma.

In addition to the neuroendocrine carcinomas, some non-small cell carcinomas without neuroendocrine morphology, especially

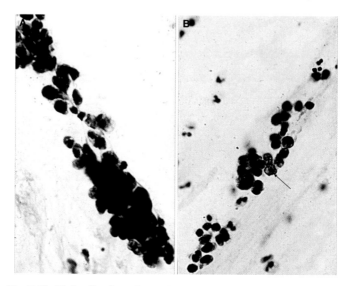

Fig. 7.48 (**A**) Small cell carcinoma. Transthoracic FNA. The neoplastic cells are slightly larger than those of a typical small cell carcinoma, but they have high nuclear/cytoplasmic ratios and lack nucleoli. (**B**) Poorly differentiated adenocarcinoma. Transthoracic FNA. The presence of the prominent, irregularly shaped nucleolus (*arrow*) separates this neoplasm from small cell carcinoma (Papanicolaou stain, medium power)

adenocarcinoma, may show neuroendocrine differentiation by immunohistochemistry. These tumors are classified according to the conventional type, with a qualifier to indicate this feature, e.g., adenocarcinoma with neuroendocrine differentiation.

Carcinoid Tumors

Carcinoid tumors, especially typical carcinoid, are usually associated with bronchi and the majority are centrally located. An endobronchial location is frequent; but because of the overlying epithelium, they usually do not exfoliate into the bronchial lumen to be detected in the secretions. In rare cases of ulcerated epithelium, and with vigorous bronchial brushing, tumor cells may be found in sputum, bronchial brush or lavage specimens. Fine needle

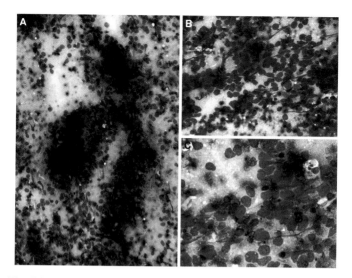

Fig. 7.49 Metastatic basaloid carcinoma mimicking small cell carcinoma. Transthoracic FNA. (**A–C**) The cytomorphologic features of this neoplasm, as shown above, are indistinguishable from those of small cell carcinoma. This patient had a history of basaloid carcinoma of the tongue and presented with multiple lung nodules. Review of the original neoplasm showed the same morphology. [Diff-Quik stain; (**A**) low power, (**B**) medium power, (**C**) high power]

aspirations, transbronchial or transthoracic depending upon the location, provide the diagnosis.

The typical carcinoid architecture, trabeculae, anastomozing cords, nests, and rosette-like formations, can be seen in cytologic preparations. Varying combinations of single or loosely cohesive cells as well as cellular tissue fragments are present (Fig. 7.51). Because of the rich vascularity of these tumors, capillaries surrounded with tumor cells can be seen in the fine needle aspirates (Fig. 7.52). Tumor cells are uniform, with round to ovoid nuclei and scant or moderate amounts of cytoplasm. Nuclei, typically, display evenly dispersed granular chromatin (Fig. 7.53). In the cellular tissue fragments, nuclear overlapping can be seen, but nuclear molding is uncommon. Some carcinoid tumors, especially

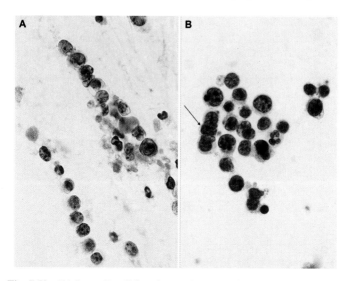

Fig. 7.50 (**A**) Large B cell lymphoma. Sputum. (**B**) Small cell carcinoma. Transbronchial FNA. Note the similarities in the selected areas of these tumors. Although there are single cells similar to those in large cell lymphoma, the presence of a short column of neoplastic cells with apparent nuclear molding (*arrow*) is diagnostic for small cell carcinoma (Papanicolaou stain, high power)

peripheral carcinoid, may have predominantly spindle cell features (Figs. 7.54 and 7.55).

Atypical carcinoid can be differentiated from typical carcinoid by the presence of focal necrosis and increased mitoses, accurate assessment of which usually requires examination of resected specimens. Cytologic specimens may show some features, such as increased cell size, suggestive of atypical carcinoid; but in our experience, a definitive specific diagnosis is not usually possible in these specimens.

Immunohistochemistry: Neuroendocrine markers, i.e., chromogranin, synaptophysin, CD56 and CD57, are strongly positive in typical carcinoid tumors (Figs. 7.56 and 7.57). Cytokeratins are positive in the majority of the tumors.

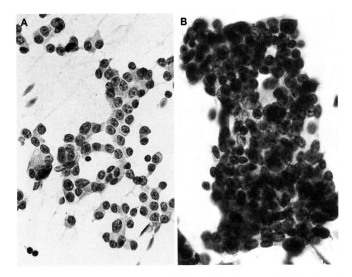

Fig. 7.51 Carcinoid tumor. (**A**) Bronchial brush. Uniform neoplastic cells with round to oval nuclei and delicate cytoplasm forming anastomozing cords. (**B**) Transthoracic FNA. A hypercellular tissue fragment of the carcinoid tumor. Note the rosette-like arrangements and crowding and overlapping of the nuclei without molding (Papanicolaou stain, high power)

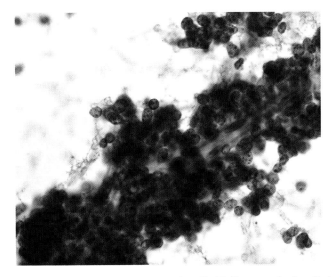

Fig. 7.52 Typical carcinoid. Transthoracic FNA. Uniform neoplastic cells in rosette-like arrangements around a capillary (Papanicolaou stain, high power)

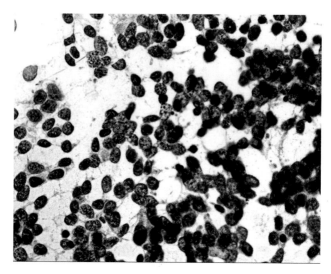

Fig. 7.53 Typical carcinoid. Transthoracic FNA. Round or ovoid nuclei with the characteristic granular chromatin (so-called "salt and pepper") pattern (Papanicolaou stain, high power)

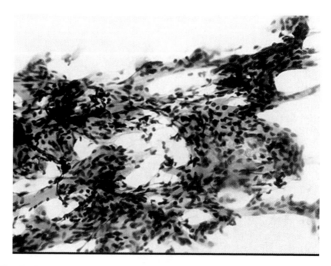

Fig. 7.54 Typical carcinoid (spindle cell type). Transthoracic FNA. A peripheral carcinoid composed of spindle cells (Papanicolaou stain, medium power)

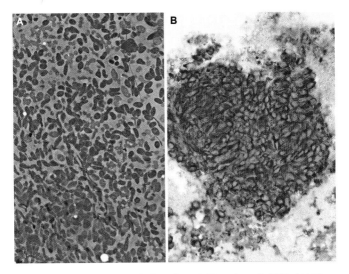

Fig. 7.55 Typical carcinoid (spindle cell type). Transthoracic FNA. (**A**) Hypercellular specimen containing predominantly elongated, spindly nuclei. (**B**) Immunoperoxidase stain for chromogranin is strongly positive. [(**A**) Diff-Quik stain, medium power; (**B**) Immunoperoxidase stain for chromogranin, medium power]

Key features: typical carcinoid

- Uniform tumor cells
- Uniform, round or oval nuclei with evenly dispersed granular chromatin
- Rosette formations
- Mitoses are absent or rare
- Immunoreactive to neuroendocrine markers

Key features: atypical carcinoid

- Tumor cells with neuroendocrine features as in typical carcinoid
- Focal necrosis and mitoses may be present

Differential diagnosis: The major differential diagnosis of typical and atypical carcinoid tumors involves other primary

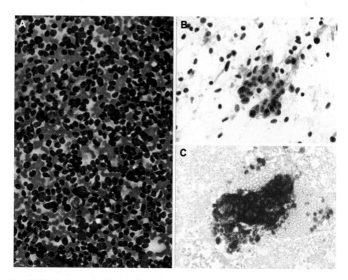

Fig. 7.56 Typical carcinoid. Transthoracic FNA. (**A**) Cellular specimen composed of predominantly single cells, small groups, and short columns. (**B**) Note the uniform round or ovoid nuclei with occasional small nucleoli. The typical granular chromatin pattern is not present. (**C**) Immunostain for chromogranin is strongly positive. [(**A**) Diff-Quik stain, medium power, (**B**) Papanicolaou stain, high power, (**C**) Immuno-peroxidase stain for chromogranin, high power]

neuroendocrine neoplasms of the lung. The presence of extensive necrosis and a high number of mitotic figures rule out carcinoid tumor. However, absence of these features in small samples, such as brushing or FNA specimens, does not rule out a high grade neuroendocrine neoplasm. Focal nuclear molding may be seen in carcinoid tumors (Fig. 7.58). Extensive molding of tumor cells with small cell features (i.e., high n/c ratio, absence of prominent nucleoli) would rule out carcinoid tumor. Clinical and radiological correlation is essential to establish the diagnosis in borderline cases.

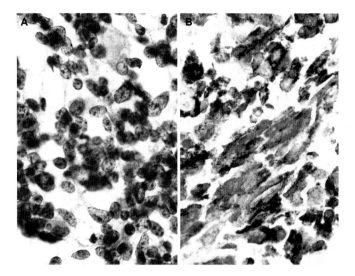

Fig. 7.57 Typical carcinoid. Transthoracic FNA. (**A**) The neoplastic cells are somewhat larger than those usually seen in typical carcinoid, and the nuclei have coarsely granular chromatin with occasional irregular clumping and delicate, ill defined cytoplasm. (**B**) The strong reaction to immunostain for chromogranin indicates the neuroendocrine nature of the tumor. Atypical carcinoid was considered, but there was no necrosis and mitoses were present. The final diagnosis of the resected tumor was typical carcinoid. [(**A**) Papanicolaou stain, high power; (**B**) Immunoperoxidase stain for chromogranin, high power]

Salivary Glandlike Tumors

Salivary glandlike tumors rarely develop in the lung, and when encountered, they are mostly encountered in the bronchi and central lung field. The most common two types seen are adenoid cystic carcinoma and mucoepidermoid carcinoma.

Adenoid Cystic Carcinoma

Adenoid cystic carcinomas comprise less than 1% of lung cancers. The majority of the tumors occur in the 4th and 5th decades of life. There is no relation to smoking tobacco products or other

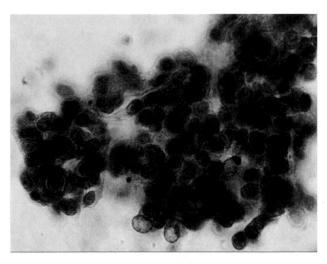

Fig. 7.58 Typical carcinoid. Transthoracic FNA. Note the focal nuclear molding. Neoplastic cells, however, have larger cytoplasm than those of small cell carcinoma (Papanicolaou stain, high power)

environmental factors. Of these tumors, 90% occur in the trachea, mainstem or lobar bronchi and present as polypoid intraluminal growths. About 20% metastasize to regional lymph nodes. Systemic metastases occur in about 40% of cases. The cytopathologic diagnosis can be made by transtracheal/bronchial fine needle aspiration or sometimes by brush specimens. On-site evaluation using Romanowsky stains (e.g., Diff-Quik) usually provides an immediate diagnosis.

Cytologically, the epithelial cells are uniform, with dark, round or oval nuclei and scant cytoplasm surrounding hyalin (basement membrane-like) globular structures. In Romanowsky stains, the globular centers stain magenta (Figs. 7.59 and 7.60).

The tumor cells show positive staining for cytokeratin as well as for myoepithelial markers (i.e., vimentin, smooth muscle actin, S-100, calponin, P 63 and CrFAP).

Differential diagnosis: In adequate samples, the tumor has distinct cytomorphology which separates it from other lung

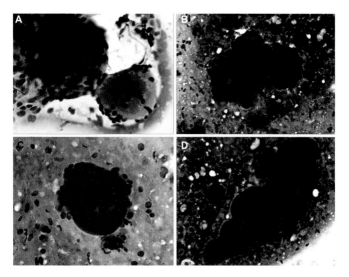

Fig. 7.59 Adenoid cystic carcinoma. Transthoracic FNA. (**A–D**) Tissue fragments of single and multiple globular structures surrounded by uniform tumor cells. Note the metachromatic staining of the globules with Diff-Quik stain. [(**A**) Papanicolaou stain, (**B–D**) Diff-Quik stain, (**A,C**) high power, (**B,D**) medium power]

tumors. Metastatic adenoid cystic carcinoma requires clinical/ radiological correlation to diagnose the metastatic nature of the tumor.

Mucoepidermoid Carcinoma

Mucoepidermoid carcinoma is a very rare tumor of the lung (less than 1% of primary lung cancers) which occurs at younger ages. About half of the patients are under 30 years old. Most of the tumors occur in the main, lobar, and segmental bronchi. Low grade tumors may involve regional lymph nodes by local invasion. Distinct metastases occur in high grade tumors.

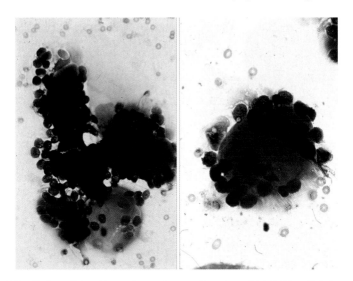

Fig. 7.60   Adenoid cystic carcinoma. Transbronchial FNA. Globular, metachromatic structure surrounded by neoplastic cells with uniform round nuclei (Diff-Quik stain, high power)

Cytologic material shows a combination of tumor cells with squamous and glandular differentiation (Fig. 7.61). In low grade tumors, mucin secreting glandular epithelium and nonkeratinizing squamous cells are identified. High grade tumors show poorly differentiated cells, mostly nonkeratinizing squamous type, and glandular epithelium may be scant.

Differential diagnosis: In limited cytologic samples, it is difficult to differentiate from squamous cell carcinoma. Peripheral tumors are usually metastatic squamous cell carcinomas. Differential diagnosis from adenosquamous carcinoma of lung is debatable, even in resected specimens. The growth pattern, absence of in situ squamous carcinoma in the overlying epithelium, absence of keratinization, and areas transitioning to low grade mucoepidermoid carcinoma are cited as criteria favoring mucoepidermoid carcinoma. Metastatic mucoepidermoid tumor can be differentiated by clinical/radiological correlation.

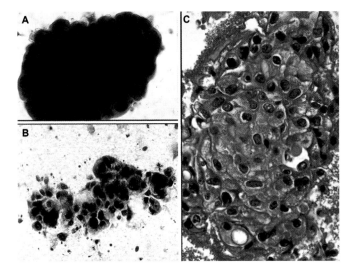

Fig. 7.61 Mucoepidermoid tumor. Transthoracic FNA. (**A**) A rounded tissue fragment with undulated borders composed of neoplastic cells with moderately increased nuclear/cytoplasmic ratios. The dense, hyaline-like appearance of the cytoplasm suggests squamous differentiation. (**B**) An aggregate of neoplastic cells with pleomorphic nuclei. No definitive features of glandular or squamous differentiation. (**C**) Tissue section from the cell block. Note the squamoid features and occasional intracytoplasmic vacuoles suggestive of glandular differentiation, which could be confirmed with mucin stains. [(**A**,**B**) Papanicolaou stain, (**C**) Hematoxylin + eosin stain, (**A**,**C**) high power, (**B**) medium power]

Suggested Reading

Alasio TM, Sun W, Yang GCH. Giant cell carcinoma of the lung impact of diagnosis and review of cytological features. Diagn Cytopathol 2007;35:555–559

Al-Haddad M, Wallace MB. EUS-FNA and biomarkers for the staging of non-small cell lung cancer. Endoscopy 2006;38:114–117

Anderson C, Ludwig ME, O'Donnell M, et al. Fine needle aspiration cytology of pulmonary carcinoid tumors. Acta Cytol 1990;34:505–510

Auger M, Katz AL, Johnston DA. Differentiating cytologic features of bronchioalveolar carcinoma from adenocarcinoma of the lung in fine-needle aspiration: a statistical analysis of 27 cases. Diagn Cytopathol 1997;16:253–257

Baba M, Iyoda A, Nomoto Y, et al. Cytological findings of pre-invasive bronchial lesions detected by light-induced fluorescence endoscopy in a lung cancer screening system. Oncol Rep 2007;17:579–583

Beasley MB. Immunohistochemistry of pulmonary and pleural neoplasia. Arch Pathol Lab Med. 2008 Jul;132:1062–1072. Review

Bhat N, Bhagat P, Pearlman ES, et al. Transbronchial needle aspiration biopsy in the diagnosis of pulmonary neoplasms. Diagn Cytopathol 1990;6:14–17

Cagle PT, Kovach M, Ramzy I. Causes of false results in transthoracic fine needle lung aspirates. Acta Cytol 1993;37:16–20

Dabbs DJ. Diagnostic immunohistochemistry, ed 2. New York, NY, Churchill Livingstone, 2002

Dacic S. EGFR assays in lung cancer. Adv Anat Pathol 2008;15:241–247. Review

Dacic S. Pulmonary preneoplasia. Arch Pathol Lab Med 2008;132:1073–1078. Review

Daneshbod Y, Modjtahedi E, Atefi S, et al. Exfoliative cytologic findings of primary pulmonary adenoid cystic carcinoma. A report of 2 cases with a review of the cytologic features. Acta Cytol 2007;51:558–562

Duncan LD, Jacob S, Atkinson S. Fine needle aspiration findings of micropapillary carcinoma in the lung. A case report. Acta Cytol 2007;51:605–608

Erkiliç S, Ozsaraç C, Küllü S. Sputum cytology for the diagnosis of lung cancer: comparison of smear and modified cell block methods. Acta Cytol 2003;47:1023–1027

Fekete PS, Cohen C, DeRose PB. Pulmonary spindle cell carcinoid-needle aspiration biopsy, histologic and histochemical findings. Acta Cytol 1990;34:50–56

Franks TJ, Galvin JR. Lung tumors with neuroendocrine morphology: essential radiologic and pathologic features. Arch Pathol Lab Med 2008 Jul;132(7):1055–1061. Review.

Herbst JB, Walts AE. High-grade neuroendocrine carcinoma presenting as an abscess: diagnosis by fine needle aspiration and review of the literature. Diagn Cytopathol 2008;36:670–673

Hiroshima K, Abe S, Ebihara Y, et al. Cytological characteristics of pulmonary large cell neuroendocrine carcinoma. Lung Cancer 2005;48:331–337

Hiroshima K, Iyoda A, Shida T, et al. Distinction of pulmonary large cell neuroendocrine carcinoma from small cell lung carcinoma: a morphological, immunohistochemical, and molecular analysis. Mod Pathol 2006;19:1358–1368

Hughes JH, Young NA, Wilber DC, et al. Cytopathology Resource Committee, College of American Pathologists: Fine-needle aspiration of pulmonary hamartoma: a common source of false-positive diagnosis in the

College of American Pathologists Interlaboratory Comparison Program in Nongynecologic Cytology. Arch Pathol Lab Med 2005;129:19–22

Kakinuma H, Mikami T, Iwabuchi K, et al. Diagnostic findings of bronchial brush cytology for pulmonary large cell neuroendocrine carcinomas: comparison with poorly differentiated adenocarcinomas, squamous cell carcinomas, and small cell carcinomas. Cancer 2003;99:247–254

Katz RL, Zaidi TM, Fernandez RL, et al. Automated detection of genetic abnormalities combined with cytology in sputum is a sensitive predictor of lung cancer. Mod Pathol 2008;21:1065

Kennedy TC, McWilliams A, Edell E, et al. American College of Chest Physicians: Bronchial intraepithelial neoplasia/early central airways lung cancer: ACCP Evidence-based Clinical Practice Guidelines (2nd ed). Chest 2007;132:221S–233S

Marek W, Richartz G, Philippou S, et al. Sputum screening for lung cancer in radon exposed uranium miners: a comparison of semi-automated sputum cytometry and conventional cytology. J Physiol Pharmacol 2007;58 Suppl 5(Pt 1):349–361

Marmor S, Koren R, Halpern M, et al. Transthoracic needle biopsy in the diagnosis of large-cell neuroendocrine carcinoma of the lung. Diagn Cytopathol 2005;33:238–243

Mathews S, Erozan YS. Pulmonary sequestration – a diagnostic pitfall. A case report. Diagn Cytopathol 1997;16:353–357

Mullins RK, Thompson SK, Coogan PS, et al. Paranuclear blue inclusions: an aid in the cytopathologic diagnosis of primary and metastatic pulmonary small-cell carcinoma. Diagn Cytopathol 1994;4:332–335

Naryshkin S, Young NA. Respiratory cytology: a review of non-neoplastic mimics of malignancy. Diagn Cytopathol 1993;9:89–97

Nicholson SA, Ryan MR. A review of cytologic findings in neuroendocrine carcinomas including carcinoid tumors with histologic correlations. Cancer Cytopathol 2000;90:148–161

Policarpio-Nicolas MLC, Wick MR. False-positive interpretations in respiratory cytopathology: exemplary cases and literature review. Diagn Cytopathol 2008;36:13–19

Saad RS, Lindner JL, Lin X et al. The diagnostic utility of D2-40 for malignant mesothelioma versus pulmonary carcinoma with pleural involvement. Diagn Cytopathol 2006;34:801–806

Saleh HA, Haapaniemi J, Khatib G, et al. Bronchioloalveolar carcinoma. Diagnostic pitfalls and immunocytochemical contribution. Diagn Cytopathol 1998;18:301–306

Shibuya K, Fujisawa T, Hoshino H, et al. Fluorescence bronchoscopy in the detection of preinvasive bronchial lesions in patients with sputum cytology suspicious or positive for malignancy. Lung Cancer 2001;32:19–25

Silverman JF, Finley JL, Park HK, et al. Fine needle aspiration cytology of bronchioloalveolar cell carcinoma of the lung. Acta Cytol 1995;29:887–894

Thiryayi SA, Rana DN, Perera DM. Bronchial carcinoid tumor: cytologic features on ThinPrep and a diagnostic pitfall in bronchial brushings and washings. Diagn Cytopathol 2008;36:275–276

Travis WD, Brambilla E, Muller-Hermelink HK, et al (eds). World Health Organization classification of tumours. Pathology and genetics of tumours of the lung, pleura, thymus and heart. IARC Press, Lyon, 2004

Wang KP, Marsh BR, Summer WR, et al. Transbronchial needle aspiration for diagnosis of lung cancer. Chest 1981;80:48–50

Wiatrowska BA, Krol J, Zakowski MF. Large-cell neuroendocrine carcinoma of the lung: proposed criteria for cytologic diagnosis. Diagn Cytopathol 2001;24:58–64

Wong PW, Stefanec T, Brown K, et al. Role of fine-needle aspirates of focal lung lesions in patients with hematologic malignancies. Chest 2002;121:527–532

Wu M, Szporn AH, Zhang D, et al. Cytology applications of p63 and TTF-1 immunostaining in differential diagnosis of lung cancers. Diagn Cytopathol 2005;33:223–227

Yang YJ, Steele CT, Ou XL, et al. Diagnosis of high-grade pulmonary neuroendocrine carcinoma by fine-needle aspiration biopsy: nonsmall-cell or small-cell type? Diagn Cytopathol 2001:25:292–300

Zaman SS, vanHoeven KH, Slott S, et al. Distinction between bronchioloalveolar carcinoma and hyperplastic pulmonary proliferations: a cytologic and morphometric analysis. Diagn Cytopathol 1997;16:396–401

Zhang H, Liu J, Cagle PT, et al. Distinction of pulmonary small cell carcinoma from poorly differentiated squamous cell carcinoma: an immunohistochemical approach. Mod Pathol 2005;18:111–118

Chapter 8
Primary Nonepithelial Malignancies

Lymphomas

Primary lymphomas of lung are rare (less than 1% of lung tumors), and the majority of them are marginal zone B-cell lymphomas of mucosa-associated lymphoid tissues (MALT) type. Diffuse large B-cell lymphomas comprise a small proportion (5–20%) of the primary lung lymphomas. Primary pulmonary Hodgkin lymphoma is very rare. Other lymphomas, Hodgkin and non-Hodgkin types, may also involve lung as part of the systemic disease.

Cytopathology

Hodgkin lymphoma, as in other sites, is diagnosed by identifying Reed-Sternberg cells, usually in transbronchial/tracheal fine needle aspirations. On rare occasions, the typical Reed-Sternberg cells can be found in sputum (Fig. 8.1A,B). Immunostains for CD30, CD15, and Fascin confirm the diagnosis (Fig. 8.2). *Low grade lymphomas*, such as MALT type which are composed mostly of small lymphocytes, are difficult to diagnose in cytologic samples, such as needle aspirations and bronchial brush or wash specimens. The diagnosis of lymphoma can be made by showing clonal B-cell populations by flow cytometry or

Y.S. Erozan, I. Ramzy, *Pulmonary Cytopathology*,
Essentials in Cytopathology 6, DOI 10.1007/978-0-387-88888-0_8,
© Springer Science+Business Media, LLC 2009

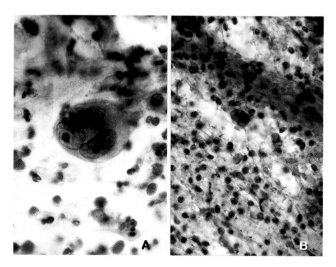

Fig. 8.1 Hodgkin lymphoma. Reed-Sternberg cells in (**A**) Sputum and (**B**) Transbronchial FNA. [Papanicolaou stain (**A**) high power, oil, ×100 objective, (**B**) high power]

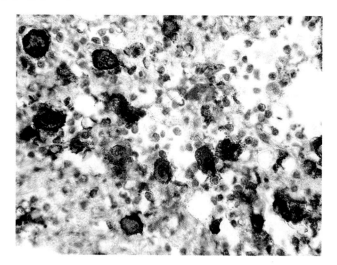

Fig. 8.2 Hodgkin lymphoma. Transbronchial FNA. Cell block. Reed-Sternberg cells in a background of lymphocytes. (Immunoperoxidase stain for CD15, high power)

immunohistochemistry in the cell blocks, if adequate specimen is available. Diagnosis of the specific type of lymphoma, however, is rarely made in these samples.

Primary diffuse large B-cell lymphomas have features typical of large cell lymphomas at other sites. Large lymphoid cells, 2–4 times the size of normal lymphocytes, have conspicuous nucleoli and express B-cell antigens (CD20, CD79a) (Fig. 8.3A,B).

Key Features: Hodgkin lymphoma
- Reed-Sternberg cells
- Positive staining with CD15, CD30 and Fascin

Key Features: MALT lymphoma
- Predominantly small lymphocytes
- Monoclonal B-cell population

Key Features: diffuse large B-cell lymphoma
- Large lymphoid cells with prominent nucleoli
- Monoclonal B-cell population

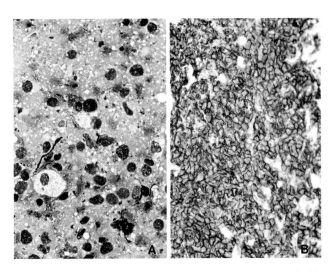

Fig. 8.3 Large B-cell lymphoma. Transthoracic FNA. (**A**) Large atypical lymphoid cells. (Compare the size with the rare small lymphocytes.) (**B**) Monoclonal, CD20 + B-cell population. [(**A**) Papanicolaou stain, high power, (**B**) Immunoperoxidase stain for CD20]

Differential diagnosis: Lymphomas should be differentiated from benign lymphocytic infiltration and proliferation, primary and metastatic small cell malignant neoplasms, neuroendocrine neoplasms, poorly differentiated carcinomas, and some sarcomas. Well differentiated lymphomas cannot be differentiated from benign lymphocytic infiltrates or reactive hyperplastic lymphoid tissue with certainty by cytomorphology alone. Phenotyping studies using flow cytometry or immunohistochemistry (in cell blocks or core biopsies) are necessary to establish the diagnosis. These methods are routinely used in all cases when a lymphoma is suspected, both for differential diagnosis from other malignancies and establishing (or confirming) the specific type. Single cell presentation of lymphomas in cytologic preparations is helpful to differentiate them from carcinomas in most cases. Some poorly differentiated adenocarcinomas, as well as some nonepithelial tumors such as melanoma, may appear entirely composed of single cells and can be difficult to differentiate morphologically from anaplastic lymphomas. Immunohistochemistry using appropriate markers establishes the diagnosis.

Sarcomas

Primary sarcomas of lung are rare; most involving the lung are metastatic. In the WHO classification, primary pulmonary sarcomas are listed as epithelioid hemangioendothelioma/angiosarcoma, sarcoma of pulmonary artery and pulmonary vein and pulmonary synovial sarcoma. Data on the cytopathologic features of these tumors are limited and mostly based on FNA specimens from extrapulmonary sites or metastatic tumors in the lung. The great majority of the cytologic samples are obtained by FNA. Definitive diagnosis of the specific type of primary sarcoma of lung usually requires a tissue specimen and ancillary techniques such as immunohistochemistry or sometimes molecular/genetic studies. Basic cytopathologic features of these tumors and their differential diagnoses from other neoplasms and non-neoplastic lesions will be discussed briefly. Examples of some of the metastatic sarcomas are illustrated in Chap. 9.

Cytopathology

FNA specimens obtained from primary sarcomas of the lung are usually very cellular. Most have spindle-cell components in varying proportions. Synovial cell sarcomas may have only spindle cells (most common type) or a mixture of epithelial and spindle cells. In most cases, the spindle cells appear in tight clusters (tissue fragments) in a background of single cells. Poorly-differentiated, high grade sarcomas tend to have predominantly or entirely single cells with anaplastic features.

Immunohisto/cytochemistry is helpful to determine the cell type. Although cytologic alcohol-fixed or air-dried preparations have been used for immunostaining with satisfactory results, sections of formalin-fixed, paraffin-embedded tissue (e.g., cell block, needle core biopsies) are preferred by many because of the well established standards for this technique. Epithelial (cytokeratins, EMA), vascular (CD31, CD34), and muscular (actin, desmin) markers are generally used.

Spindle-cell sarcomas react to markers according to their specific type. Synovial cell sarcomas generally react to both cytokeratins, especially CK-7 and CK-9, and EMA. This reactivity is seen in both spindle cell and epithelial cell components, but stronger in the latter. The spindle cell component is reactive for vimentin, and about one third of synovial cell sarcomas are reactive to S-100 (nuclear and cytoplasmic staining). In some of the synovial sarcomas, other techniques, such as FISH, are needed to demonstrate the characteristic chromosomal changes, translocation between X and 18 chromosomes, to establish the diagnosis.

Key Features
- Very cellular material
- Most have spindle cells in varying proportions
- Synovial sarcomas may have only spindle cells or a mixed epithelial and spindle cell component
- Poorly differentiated high-grade sarcomas tend to have predominantly single cells with anaplastic features

Differential diagnosis: Primary sarcomas of lung should be differentiated from benign spindle cell lesions, spindle cell carcinomas of lung, metastatic sarcomas, and carcinomas with spindle cell features.

Benign spindle cell neoplasms in the lung are extremely rare. Solitary fibrous tumor is a neoplasm of pleura and can be distinguished radiologically from intrapulmonary spindle cell sarcomas.

Inflammatory myofibroblastic tumor may have predominantly spindle cell component in FNA specimens, but the presence of inflammatory cell component, lymphocytes, plasma cells and histiocytes differentiates this tumor from spindle cell sarcomas.

Healing pneumonias and granulomas may also have a predominant spindle cell component, but other elements, such as chronic inflammatory cells, histiocytes, and reactive pneumocytes are also present in these lesions.

Primary sarcomatoid carcinomas have varying proportions of spindle cell components. Immunostain for cytokeratins and EMA may help in the differential diagnosis, except for synovial sarcomas. Pure spindle cell carcinoma does not react to antibodies for cytokeratin and EMA. Differentiating this tumor from spindle cell sarcoma is very difficult, if not impossible.

Carcinoid tumor with spindle cells can be differentiated by its positive staining with neuroendocrine markers. Differential diagnosis between primary sarcomas and their counterparts which metastasize to lung can only be made with clinical and radiological correlation.

Suggested Reading

Hummel P, Cangiarella JF, Cohen JM, et al. Transthoracic fine-needle aspiration biopsy of pulmonary spindle cell and mesenchymal lesions: a study of 61cases. Cancer (Cancer Cytopathol) 2001;93:187–198

Kumar R, Sidhu H, Mistry R, et al. Primary pulmonary Hodgkin's lymphoma: a rare pitfall in transthoracic fine needle aspiration cytology. Diagn Cytopathol 2008;36:666–669

Litzky LA. Pulmonary sarcomatous tumors. Arch Pathol Lab Med.2008; 132:1104–1117. Review

Weiss SW, Goldblum JR. Enzinger and Weiss's Soft Tissue Tumors, ed 5, Philadelphia, PA, Elsevier, 2008

Chapter 9
Metastatic Tumors

The development of pulmonary metastases is one of the most common findings in late stages of malignancies. Autopsy studies demonstrate metastasis in 50–100% of patients with a wide variety of malignancies. The relative incidence of the primary sites reflects changing epidemiology of various cancers over time and across geographic locations. In North America, as an example, breast is the most common source; in the Far East the majority originates in the gastrointestinal tract. In women, the most likely source of hematogenous spread is the breast, ovary, colon, and mesenchymal malignancies, while in men, the colon, kidney and testis are often the source. Lymphangitic spread is responsible for about 7% of lung metastases, and almost all such tumors are adenocarcinomas originating from breast, gastrointestinal tract, prostate, pancreas, ovary and lung.

Metastatic lesions usually present as multiple nodules, but in 1–5% of cases a solitary mass is encountered, particularly in carcinomas of breast, colon, bladder, and kidney as well as in melanomas and sarcomas. Cytology offers a spectrum of noninvasive sampling modalities to establish or confirm the diagnosis of metastatic tumors. Surgical open biopsy or excision is reserved for cases lacking history or clinical evidence of an extrapulmonary primary, or when there is a possibility of improved survival following resection of solitary metastases. Such improved outcome has been reported to benefit some patients with carcinomas of breast, colon, renal cell carcinoma, melanoma and sarcoma.

Y.S. Erozan, I. Ramzy, *Pulmonary Cytopathology*,
Essentials in Cytopathology 6, DOI 10.1007/978-0-387-88888-0_9,
© Springer Science+Business Media, LLC 2009

Table 9.1 Determining primary site and type of cancer

History of previous tumor
Clinical and radiological findings
Cytomorphology and comparison with previous tumor, if available
Ancillary techniques
  – Special stains (e.g., stains for mucin)
  – Immunohisto/cytochemistry
  – Flow cytometry
  – Molecular/genetic techniques
  – Electron microscopy

The efficacy of each modality of cytologic sampling depends on the location, size, anatomic relations and availability of technical expertise. It is enhanced by the judicial use of ancillary techniques (Table 9.1). The usual route for metastases to the lung is via blood in the form of tumor emboli. These settle in small vessels and in early stages have no connection to bronchi, thus they are unlikely to be detected in sputum, bronchial brushings, lavage or biopsies. Eventually, tumors invade the submucosal lymphatics in the bronchial wall and neoplastic cells may appear in sputum or bronchial brush/lavage specimens. Diagnostic material may be procured by FNA if a mass is visualized by one of the imaging techniques. Endobronchial metastasis to the bronchial wall may develop, particularly in cases of renal cell and colonic carcinomas, and as such can yield diagnostic cells in sputum and bronchial brushing samples.

Differential Diagnosis: General Considerations

Metastatic disease in patients with known primary is usually detected on followup imaging studies. However, unsuspected metastases can be the first indication of malignancy, appearing in the form of single or multiple nodules, or mediastinal widening on imaging. In other instances, the clinical scenario simulates interstitial, inflammatory, obstructive or other nonneoplastic pulmonary diseases, as listed below. Occlusion of a large number of small arteries by tumor emboli results in pulmonary hypertension; spread via lymphatics in septa and subpleura produces an interstitial disease-like pattern. Some cases present with respiratory insufficiency or bronchial obstruction and its sequelae. The role of cytology in clarifying the neoplastic nature within these scenarios, and the selection of the appropriate technique, depend on the nature of the infiltrate and its location. A multidisciplinary approach and an open communication with the pulmonologist and radiologist are of paramount importance.

Atypical presenting features of metastatic lung tumors

- Interstitial pneumonia-like
- Pulmonary hypertension
- Cavitary lesion, cyst or abscess
- Bronchial obstruction
- Respiratory insufficiency
- Pleural thickening

Due to its vascularity, a wide spectrum of epithelial and mesenchymal malignant neoplasms reaches the lung. Most of these are adenocarcinomas; others include tumors of squamous, urothelial, neuroendocrine, mesenchymal, glial or multipotent differentiation, such as germ cell neoplasms. A detailed discussion of the cytologic features of all these tumors is beyond the scope of this text; a differential diagnostic approach to the morphologic types/patterns encountered more frequently by the practicing pathologist appears to be more appropriate.

Adenocarcinoma

This is the most common type of pulmonary metastases. The presence of multiple lesions favors the neoplasm being metastatic, although bronchioloalveolar carcinomas are often multicentric. The availability of treatment modalities tailored for different tumors puts a demand on the cytopathologist to differentiate primary from metastatic adenocarcinoma and to determine the source of the metastasis. Cytomorphologic features, enhanced by immunocytochemical studies, often help in achieving this goal. In performing ancillary stains, it is always preferable to use a sensitive screening test in addition to a specific confirming test to cover all possible diagnoses. Due to limited material, however, such luxury is not always feasible unless a cell-rich paraffin block is available, thus the need for judicial selection of stains to save valuable sample material and resources.

Adenocarcinomas can be grouped into five morphologic patterns: acinar, papillary, mucinous, solid and clear cell. Each of these raises a group of differential diagnostic issues that form the basis for the discussion followed in this chapter.

Cytomorphologic patterns of adenocarcinoma in lung
- Acinar
- Papillary
- Mucinous and signet ring cell
- Solid
- Clear cell

Adenocarcinomas with Acinar Pattern

These tumors are often of colorectal, pancreatobiliary or pulmonary origin (Fig. 9.1). The cells are tall columnar, and have elongated basally located nuclei. Marked nuclear pleomorphism favors metastasis over primary lung cancers. Acinar formations may be seen together with isolated cells and solid nests. Colonic tumors are more likely to produce "dirty" central necrosis, thus the presence of eosinophilic homogeneous material in the aspirate favors a colonic type. Colonic cells tend to be tall, with palisaded elongated "cigar-shaped" nuclei and apical mucin. Identification of focal squamous differentiation supports pancreatic or pulmonary origin of the metastasis. In the case of prostatic metastases, the cells have central nuclei with central prominent nucleoli. Immunocytochemistry can be helpful in narrowing the possibilities of origin of such metastases (Fig. 9.2). The main immunocytochemical profiles of common metastatic tumors presenting with acinar glandular pattern are summarized in Table 9.2

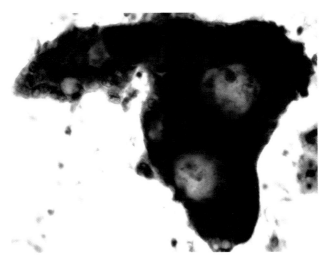

Fig. 9.1 Metastatic colon cancer. The malignant cells show two well formed acini (Papanicolaou, medium power)

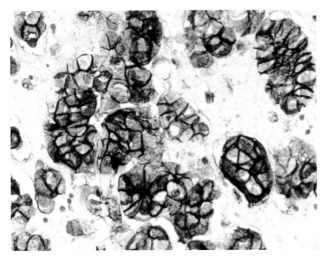

Fig. 9.2 Metastatic lung carcinoma. Positive immunoreactivity to Ber-Ep4 speaks against the tumor being a mesothelioma (Ber-Ep4, high power)

Table 9.2 Immunoprofiles of tumors with acinar formations

	TTF	CK7	CK20	CEA	BRST2	Other
Lung	±[a]	+	−	+	−	PE 10+
Colorectal	−	−	+	+	−	CA19–9 usually +
Pancreas	−	+	+	+	−	CA19–9, (amylase in acinic)
Ovary, serous	−	+	−	− (most)	−	CA125, ER
Breast	−	+	−	Variable	+	ER, PR
Prostate	−	−	−	−	−	PSA, PAP

[a]TTF immunoreactivity is seen in 70–75% of adenocarcinomas, small cell carcinomas and large cell neuroendocrine carcinomas are immunoreactive to TTF, but only in 10% of squamous cell carcinomas and 25% of large cell carcinomas.

Adenocarcinomas with Mucinous/Signet-Ring Cell Pattern

These tumors often originate from breast, lung or stomach. Differentiation between primary and metastatic neoplasms is particularly difficult in view of the overlapping cytomorphologic features. A clean background around aggregates of neoplastic cells favors metastasis, although this is not a constant feature. The mucinous background may be sparsely cellular, and in bronchial lavage material, it may be difficult to identify the few malignant cells within the abundant mucinous pools in the background.

Isolated signet ring cells may be encountered, in addition to some sheets of mucinous cells with basal or central nuclei (Fig. 9.3). The cytologic features of primary bronchioloalveolar carcinoma have been discussed in detail earlier in this text (Chap. 7). These include large amounts of mucus, in which tight clusters of mucinous cells may be identified. Psammoma bodies are occasionally seen. Metastatic adenocarcinomas from extrapulmonary sites can spread along alveolar septa in a similar fashion to bronchioloalveolar carcinomas, and can secrete abundant mucus; thus the cytologic and histologic features can overlap. Colonic adenocarcinoma has a necrotic background and the cells stain negatively for TTF 1 and PE 10 surfactant antibody. Gastric and

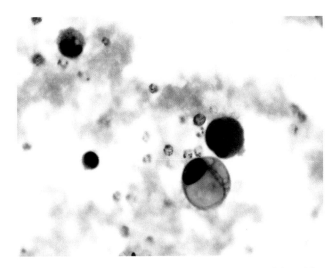

Fig. 9.3 Metastatic signet ring adenocarcinoma. This tumor originated from a gastric primary (Papanicolaou, oil, ×100 objective)

mammary carcinomas may show signet ring cells, an uncommon finding in bronchioloalveolar carcinomas, particularly in FNA specimens. The reciprocal CK7 and CK 20 staining pattern helps in differentiating lung from colonic adenocarcinomas, but not from gastric and pancreatic carcinomas which have a variable immunoreactivity to CK7 and CK20. The immunoprofiles of tumors associated with mucinous or signet ring cells are summarized in Table 9.3.

Table 9.3 Immunoprofiles of mucinous tumors

	TTF	CK7	CK20	mCEA	ER/PR	BRST2	Other
Lung	+	+	−	+	−	−	PE10+
Breast	−	+	−	Variable	+	+	EMA+
Colon	−	−	+	+	−	−	
Stomach	−	+ (most)	+	+	−	−	CA19-9
Ovary, mucinous	−	+	+	Rare	+		CA125

Carcinomas with Papillary Pattern

These are usually of pulmonary, ovarian or colonic origin. We have encountered some examples of metastatic papillary thyroid and renal cell cancers in the lung. Regardless of their origin, these tumors have elongated cells with somewhat densely eosinophilic cytoplasm, and may show psammoma bodies (Fig. 9.4; also see Fig. 2.14). Thyroid carcinomas may show the characteristic nuclear features such as nuclear folds, powdery chromatin and intranuclear cytoplasmic inclusions. The presence of psammoma bodies supports this diagnosis only in the presence of the characteristic nuclear features, since these calcified bodies are also seen in ovarian and bronchioloalveolar carcinomas. Immunoreactivity for TTF is seen in thyroid as well as in lung tumors, but immunoreactivity to thyroglobulin is limited to papillary and follicular carcinomas of the thyroid and not lung tumors.

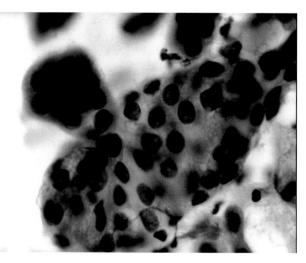

Fig. 9.4   Metastatic adenocarcinoma, papillary pattern. This tumor was of a renal cell origin. The diagnosis was supported by cytomorphologic and immunohistochemical similarity with the original papillary renal cell carcinoma. (Papanicolaou, oil, ×100 objective)

Serous ovarian carcinomas tend to have highly pleomorphic nuclei, particularly by the time they reach the late stages with development of metastases. There is a tendency for psammoma bodies to be more prominent in ovarian serous carcinomas in pulmonary or thyroid tumors. A positive staining for CA 125 and negative staining for TTF help identify these tumors. Finally, colonic carcinoma can appear as papillary formations, particularly in sputum specimens, but these are usually associated with some mucinous or acinar cells as previously discussed. Table 9.4 contrasts the immunophenotypes of papillary neoplasms.

Carcinomas with Solid Nest or Diffuse Pattern

These tumors present to the cytopathologist as solid nests or diffuse sheets of neoplastic cells, in addition to isolated cells. In the absence of a known primary for comparison, the diagnosis is often a matter of excluding common sources by a combination of morphologic and immunocytochemical profiles, as outlined in other parts of this chapter. Among the most common in this group is adenocarcinoma of breast origin, which appears as small cohesive, tightly clustered cells with nuclear molding (Fig. 9.5A, B). The characteristic single file arrangement of small cells may be seen but only in sputum specimens. Other adenocarcinomas, as well as undifferentiated tumors, often produce solid nests or clusters of isolated cells (Fig. 9.6). The differential diagnosis also encompasses melanomas, undifferentiated large cell carcinoma, squamous cell carcinoma, hepatocellular carcinoma, urothelial

Table 9.4 Immunoprofiles of tumors with papillary pattern

	TTF	Thyroglobulin	mCEA	CA 125	BRST2	Other
Lung	+	−	+	−	−	ER−
Thyroid	+	+	−	−	−	vimentin
Ovary, serous	−	−	−	+	−	ER/PR+
Breast	−	−	Variable	+	+	ER/PR+

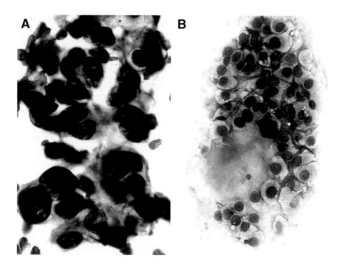

Fig. 9.5 Adenocarcinoma, metastatic from a breast primary. (**A**) Although the tumor appears mostly as solid sheets, there is a subtle tendency to form glands (Papanicolaou, oil, ×100 objective). (**B**) Chondroblastic metaplasia, seen in some breast carcinomas, is depicted in this aspirate from a patient with breast cancer (Diff-Quik, high power)

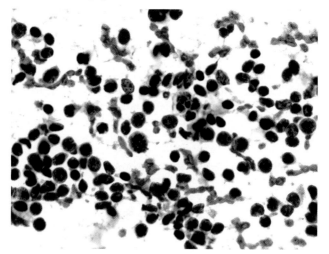

Fig. 9.6 Metastatic "small blue cell" tumor: The small cells were aspirated from the left upper lobe of a 2-year-old boy who had a neuroblastoma. The diagnosis was confirmed by immunohistochemistry (H & E, high power)

carcinoma and neuroendocrine carcinoma, as well as epithelioid sarcoma.

Tumors with Clear Cells

The differential diagnosis of clear cell tumors includes benign clear cell tumor, clear cell adenocarcinoma of the lung, renal cell carcinoma, ovarian cancer, clear cell sarcomas (e.g. of tendon sheath) and testicular tumors.

Renal cell carcinoma is much more frequently encountered in the lung than pulmonary clear cell tumor or clear cell carcinoma. The neoplastic cells have central macronucleoli and the cytoplasm is often clear due to the abundance of glycogen and lipids, hence the positive staining with PAS and Oil Red O (Fig. 9.7). Some cells, however, have granular cytoplasm, particularly in material procured by FNA. Renal cell carcinoma is immunoreactive to CD10, RCC, EMA, LMW keratins (such

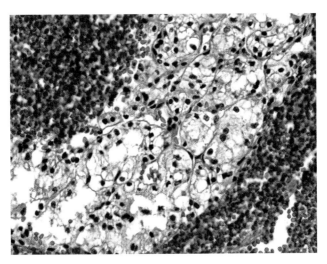

Fig. 9.7 Metastatic clear cell carcinoma. The patient had a history of renal cell carcinoma, clear cell type. Cell block preparation from an FNA (H & E, high power)

Table 9.5 Immunoprofiles of tumors with clear cells

	TTF	Ker	Vim	HMB 45	EMA	Other
Lung, clear cell benign[a]		–	+	+	–	+actin, S100, –CEA,
Carcinoma	+	+	–	–	+	α1 antichymo-trypsin
Renal	–	+LMW	+	–	+	+RCC, CD10, Oil red O, -CEA
Ovary	–	+	–	–	+	+CA125
Testis[b]	–	Variable	Variable	–	–	PLAP

[a]Benign clear cell tumor of lung and metastatic clear cell sarcoma of tendon sheath have similar immunophenotype. Clear cell carcinoma of the lung is rare
[b]HPLAP is seen in germ cell tumors, CAM 5.2 in non-seminomatous tumors; non-germ cell are CEA– but reactive to inhibin

as CAM 5.2) and vimentin. They are negative for TTF-1, CEA, inhibin, and HMB 45. Clear cell lung tumors (sugar tumor) and clear cell sarcoma of tendon sheath, in contrast, are negative for keratin and RCC, but positive for vimentin and HMB 45. Lung tumors are also immunoreactive to TTF-1. Clear cell tumors of the ovary are immunoreactive for cytokeratin and CA125. Adrenocortical carcinoma is a rare source of metastatic clear cells that should be considered. Table 9.5 summarizes the immunophenotypes of the common clear cell neoplasms.

Squamous and Transitional Cell Carcinoma

Squamous cell cancer is the most common primary lung cancer. In elderly patients with history of head and neck squamous cell carcinoma, the detection of malignancy in pulmonary specimens may still reflect the development of a new lung primary rather than metastasis, since there is an overlap of risk factors for both types of cancer. Metastasis with squamous differentiation may originate from the head and neck, lung, pancreas, cervix and occasionally in other organs. Rarely, squamous epithelium may develop as a

Table 9.6 Immunoprofiles of tumors with solid poorly differentiated pattern[a]

	AE1/AE3	CK7	CK20	CEA	EMA	S100
Urothelial (Transitional)	+	+	+	+	+	−
Squamous	+	20%	−	50%	+	−
Melanoma	−	−	−	−	−	+

[a]Other than adenocarcinoma

result of metaplastic change in the wall of a cavitating sarcomatous nodule; in such case it can present a diagnostic problem for the cytopathologist encountering atypical squamous cells in a clinical/imaging scenario of lung malignancy. Unlike metastatic tumors originating in the cervix, primary lung squamous cancers lack DNA evidence of high risk HPV, a feature which can be helpful in deciding if the lung tumor is a new primary.

Urothelial (transitional cell) carcinoma usually originates from the bladder, although some cases were reported from the cervix and upper urinary tract. The polygonal or pyramidal cells have similar cytologic features to the primary tumor, with dense, often vacuolated, cyanophilic cytoplasm. These cells also share many morphologic and immunophenotypic characteristics with poorly or moderately differentiated squamous cell carcinoma. Some of the features that differentiate these from other malignancies are listed in Table 9.6. The tumors are immunoreactive to keratins (CK7 and CK20), and to CEA, but are negative for vimentin.

Spindle Cell and Miscellaneous Nonepithelial Neoplasms

Some tumors are predominantly associated with spindle cell morphology. Such metastases usually originate from sarcomas, spindle cell carcinomas, melanomas, mesotheliomas as well as germ cell neoplasms. Table 9.7 lists some immunostains that help in the initial differentiation between the major groups of tumors in the lung. The sarcoma group includes leiomyosarcoma, endometrial

Table 9.7 Immunoprofiles of tumors with spindle cells

	Vim	Melan A	CEA	Keratin	Calretinin	Other
Melanoma	−	+	−	−	−	HMB 45, S 100
Sarcoma	+	−	−	−	−	Stromal markers e.g. MSA, etc.
Carcinoma	±	−	±	+	−	
Mesothe-lioma	+	−	−	+	+	Thrombomo-dulin, HBME 1

stromal sarcoma, MFH, angiosarcoma and synovial sarcoma (Figs. 9.8 to 9.10). The spectrum of soft tissue neoplasms is quite broad and the reader is referred to other texts for a detailed discussion of their immunocytochemical profiles (Weiss and Goldblum).

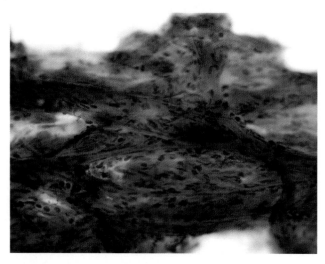

Fig. 9.8 Metastatic leiomyosarcoma. An FNA revealed the presence of this three dimensional tissue fragment. Focusing at different levels using higher magnification helps to visualize nuclear features of the neoplastic cells in such thick fragments. (Papanicolaou, medium power)

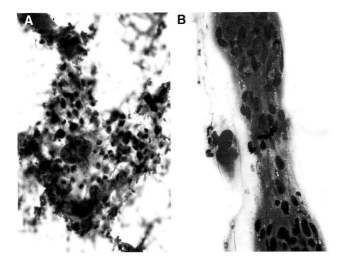

Fig. 9.9 Metastatic leiomyosarcoma. (**A**) Note the large bizarre nuclei near the center of the figure. Multinucleation and the presence of spindled cells with bizarre nuclei favor the diagnosis of a sarcoma rather than carcinoma (Papanicolaou, medium power). (**B**) An air-dried preparation showing some spindled cells. Immunocytochemical stains are almost always necessary to further classify these spindle cell neoplasms, since the cytomorphologic features of several sarcomas overlap (Diff-Quik, high power)

However, a review of the features of melanoma, a common source of pulmonary metastases, and of germ cell tumors is appropriate.

M*etastatic melanoma* can be difficult to diagnose if the tumor is nonpigmented, since the cytomorphology can be similar to large cell undifferentiated malignancy. Clues to the nature of this biphasic tumor include a mixture of polygonal and spindled cells with abundant cytoplasm that is usually cyanophilic and may contain granules that stain greenish brown with Papanicoloaou stain (Fig. 9.11). The nuclei posses macronucleoli, and often contain intranuclear cytoplasmic vacuoles. Binucleation is frequently encountered in these cells. Immunoreactivity to S100 protein is a sensitive, but not specific test for identifying melanoma; more specific stains such as Melan A or HMB 45 are needed to confirm the diagnosis.

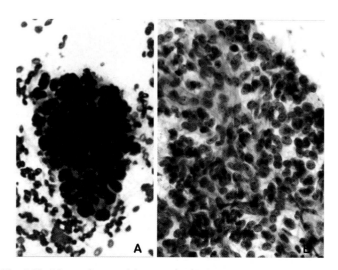

Fig. 9.10 Metastatic synovial sarcoma. (**A**) A cellular aspirate with a cell aggregate showing nuclear pleomorphism and high nuclear cytoplasm ratio (Diff-Quik, high power). (**B**) The epithelial like cells show some tendency to gland differentiation and are mixed with a few spindle cells. The dual cell population helps to narrow the differential diagnosis, but immunohistochemistry is necessary to support the diagnosis (Papanicolaou, intermediate power)

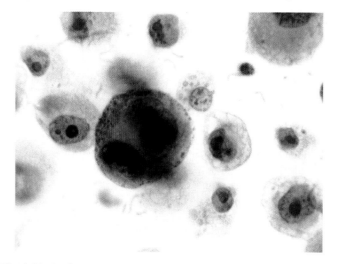

Fig. 9.11 Malignant melanoma, metastatic. Note the prominent nucleoli, multinucleation and the pigment granules in the cytoplasm (Papanicolaou, oil, ×100 objective)

Key features of metastatic amelanotic melanoma
- Many isolated cells
- Abundant cytoplasm, polygonal and/or spindled
- Binucleation
- Intranuclear cytoplasmic vacuoles
- Prominent nucleoli with perinucleolar clearing
- Immunoreactivity to S 100, Melan A, HMB 45

Germ cell tumors are nonepithelial or multipotent neoplasms that occasionally metastasize to the lungs or develop as primary lesions in the mediastinum. Their cells cover a spectrum of epithelial like to spindle morphology, with marked cytologic and nuclear pleomorphism and hyperchromasia; they can be correctly identified if there is a history of a testicular or ovarian primary, as well as by demonstration of α-fetoprotein or hCG immunoreactivity. These tumors encompass choriocarcinoma, embryonal carcinoma, and yolk sac tumors. Choriocarcinomas have a tendency to spread by blood and develop as multiple "cannon ball" pulmonary metastases. The diagnosis in such cases is made through assessment of hCG serum levels, and cytology is rarely needed. The lesions are hemorrhagic, and the diagnostic pleomorphic cells with abundant cytoplasm surrounding large, hyperchromatic and pleomorphic nuclei, are rarely detected.

Pleural Metastases

Metastatic deposits reach the pleura via lymphatics or blood vessels. They are more likely to yield diagnostic material by cytologic examination of pleural effusions than by biopsy of the nodules, particularly if the cytologic examination is repeated. Differentiating metastases from mesothelioma is a critical issue, but a detailed discussion of fluid cytology is beyond the scope of this text.

Concluding Remarks

The pathologist, faced with increased demand for a definitive diagnosis of tumors metastatic to the lung can be helped by a detailed history, an open three way communication with the radiologist and clinician, and careful evaluation of cytomorphologic criteria, with comparison to the original material sampled from the primary, if available. Some tumors will lend themselves easier than others, particularly with the use of ancillary studies and immunocytochemistry as depicted in Table 9.8. In other cases, the best we can offer is excluding some tumors, thus helping to narrow the differential diagnoses to be considered by the treating physician. The evolution of ancillary techniques will continue to change the landscape in this dynamic field and enhance our ability to further classify tumors that are presently designated as poorly differentiated or undifferentiated large tumors, thus helping us to tailor their treatment to improve the outcome for patients with metastatic disease in the lung.

Table 9.8   Positive immunoreactivity of common metastatic adenocarcinomas

Breast	BRST2, ER, PR, CK7 (with negative CK20), S100 and MC5
Colon	CEA, CK20 (with negative CK7)
Stomach	CK 7 and CK20
Kidney, clear cell	CD10, RCC, erythropoietin, LMW Ker (CAM 5.2), EMA, PAS and Oil Red O
Prostate	PSA and PAP
Thyroid	Follicular and papillary: TTF, Thyroglobulin, T3, T4, co express vimentin and keratin
	Medullary: neuroendocrine markers and calcitonin
Pancreas	Ductal carcinoma: CK7 and CK20
	Acinar cell carcinoma: amylase
	Islet cell tumors: neuroendocrine markers and keratin
Ovary	Epithelial non mucinous: CA125, CK7, CEA and EMA
	Epithelial mucinous: CK7, CK20, CEA, CA 125, ER and PR
	Sex cord/stroma: Inhibin, CD99
Hepatocellular	Hepar 1 (HCC), CEA (laminar), AFP
Salivary	Acinic carcinoma: amylase, a-1 antichymotrypsin
	Adenoid cystic carcinoma: S100, LMW keratin (CAM 5.2). vimentin

Suggested Reading

Chhieng DC, Cangiarella JF, Zakowski MF, et al. Use of thyroid transcription factor 1, PE-10, and cytokeratins 7 and 20 in discriminating between primary lung carcinomas and metastatic lesions in fine-needle aspiration biopsy specimens. Cancer 2001;93:330–336

Crosby JH, Hoeg K, Hager B. Transthoracic fine needle aspiration of primary and metastatic sarcomas. Diagn Cytopathol 1985;1:221–227

Dabbs DJ. Diagnostic immunohistochemistry, ed 2. Philadelphia, PA, Churchill Livingstone, 2006

Zeppa P, Cozzolino I, Russo M, et al. Pulmonary Langerhans cell Histiocytosis (Histiocytosis X) on bronchoalveolar lavage: a report of 2 cases. Acta Cytol 2007;51:480–486

Index

Printed in the United States of America